ROCKING
the PINK

Finding Myself on the
Other Side of Cancer

Laura Roppé

SEAL PRESS

Rocking the Pink
Finding Myself on the Other Side of Cancer

Copyright © 2012 by Laura Roppé

Published by
Seal Press
A Member of the Perseus Books Group
1700 Fourth Street
Berkeley, California

Library of Congress Cataloging-in-Publication Data

Roppé, Laura, 1970-
  Rocking the pink : finding my rock star self on the other side of cancer / Laura Roppé.
    p. cm.
  ISBN 978-1-58005-417-1 (paperback)
  1. Roppé, Laura, 1970—Health. 2. Breast—Cancer—Patients—Biography. I. Title.
  RC280.B8R66 2012
  362.196'994490092—dc23
  [B]
                                        2011027014

9 8 7 6 5 4 3 2 1

Cover and interior design by Domini Dragoone
Printed in the United States of America
Distributed by Publishers Group West

For Brad, my love.
For Sophie, my compass.
For Chloe, my future coconspirator.

Throughout the telling of this story, Laura Roppé references several of her self-penned songs, either as a plot point or as a lyrical window into her thoughts in a particular situation. To find out how to download some of Laura's music for free, go to www.rockingthepink.com.

Chapter 1

On a sunny morning in mid-October 2008, a whiplash-inducing phone call from my surgeon hijacked my life to the hinterlands of hell. It was a startling reversal of fortune: That very day, the *Los Angeles Daily Journal* had featured a two-page article about me entitled "In the Long Run, San Diego Lawyer Decides to Face the Music," and I was squealing with delight as I devoured every complimentary word. The article detailed how I'd been inspired to follow my midlife musical dreams after running my first full marathon.

I'd had an implausible stretch of good luck since I'd released my album two months earlier—my new record label was about to fly me to England to shoot a music video!—and now here was my elated face, smack on the front page of a respected newspaper. The photo was flattering, thankfully—my Jay Leno chin was barely noticeable as my body leaned over the impressive control panel in the recording studio.

I reached for the phone, bursting at the seams to share this triumph with my husband, Brad.

Just as I was about to dial, my surgeon called.

Oh, yeah, that whole thing.

Three days earlier, mostly to placate Brad, I'd gone in for a biopsy of an "almost certainly" benign lump in my left breast. I wasn't alarmed. I knew I didn't have *cancer.* Even uttering the C-word sounded melodramatic, like an attention-seeking stunt. I was only thirty-seven, and there was no history of the disease in my family. Plus, I'd just run a marathon, for Pete's sake.

"Oh, hi, Doc," I greeted him. "How are you?" I paused, expecting to hear his relieved chuckle.

"Laura," the doctor began. He wasn't chuckling. My stomach lurched unexpectedly as he cleared his throat. "I've got some bad news . . . "

I didn't recognize my own voice as I let out a rasping wail. My legs gave way, and I collapsed onto the couch.

The doctor was still talking. His words came to me in fragments, as if he had bad cell phone reception: " . . . down to my office right away . . . treatment plan . . . so sorry . . . "

My brain was melting down. Had he just used the word "cancer"? About *me?*

Brad. That was all I could think, over and over again. I struggled to remember his phone number at work, a number I'd called a million times. I finally got through and heard his familiar, unsuspecting voice.

"Brad," I gasped. My voice sounded garbled and foreign to me.

"Babe, can I call you right back? I've got to—"

"It's *cancer, Buddy.* Come home!" I was bawling. "Come home. *Right now!*" I was shrieking.

"I'm on my way," he said, panic raging underneath his controlled voice.

I couldn't remember who I'd been before I loved Brad. I had to go way back—to memories of losing a tooth or hanging Duran Duran posters on my bedroom walls—to conjure a firm recollection of my pre-Brad self. I'd met him twenty-three years earlier, at a summer party when I was fourteen years old, though I'd lied and said I was fifteen. Not the best way to start off one's relationship with a future spouse, but who knew I was meeting my future husband at fourteen years old? And, in my defense, I was just two months shy of my birthday, so I was *practically* fifteen.

Brad was sixteen years old, and in the prime of health and fitness, when I first laid eyes on him. He had just competed in a triathlon, and he had the eight-pack abs to prove it. He stood six feet, four inches tall and had blond hair and blue eyes—a classic California surfer boy. He would have caught any girl's eye. Except mine. No, I didn't notice Brad at first, because I had my eye on an age-inappropriate lifeguard at the party (who, to his credit, wasn't the least bit interested in a fourteen-year-old child). While my boy-crazy eye was trained on that curly-haired lifeguard, Brad approached and invited me to walk on the beach. I figured, why not?

As we ambled along the waterline, I noticed his wildly patterned, electric blue, baggy pants.

"I like your pants," I said in earnest.

"Thanks. My grandma made 'em for me."

Well, that was adorable. And sort of . . . rogue, in a perverse way. And, coincidentally, that very night, I was sporting bright yellow shorts dotted with pineapples, paired with a mismatched Hawaiian shirt—my own way of railing against the ubiquitous preppy look of the day. We looked good together, in a Jackson Pollock sort of way.

Brad was a year ahead of me in school. He'd been class president. And he loved to surf and spearfish. *Spearfish? Like Christopher Atkins in The Blue Lagoon?* He told me my brown eyes were hypnotizing him. I blushed.

"Are your parents married?" I asked, changing the subject.

"Divorced. When I was nine. I live with my dad and brother."

"Mine, too. When I was seven. I live with my mom and sister." Our symmetry was obvious. We just *fit*.

Out of sheer glee, I spontaneously rolled down a sand dune on the beach, just for the fun of it. He thought that was funny, and he let out a silly, high-pitched laugh that cracked me up. And then he kissed me, and the resulting tingles shot all the way down to my toes. An hour of talking and kissing later, Brad asked, "Can I give you a lift home in my 'Vette?"

"Sounds great."

When we had reached Brad's car, a short distance away, I was surprised to find a worn-out, steel gray Chevy Chevette sitting in front of me. "Nice 'Vette," I giggled. This was not the sparkling Corvette I had envisioned. And that suited me just fine. Considerably charmed, I got into the car.

After Brad had dropped me off at home, I crawled into bed, exhausted but floating on cloud nine. Five minutes later, before I could even drift off to sleep, my phone rang. It was Brad, calling to say good night, a romantic gesture in the age before cell phones.

"Can I see you tomorrow?" Brad wanted to know.

"Of course." I smiled into the phone. "Good night."

Who on earth has her actual, handwritten diary from the day she met her future husband, at age fourteen? Well, I do. I must be one of, like, seven people in the history of the world. At any rate, my diary entry from August 20, 1985, states:

> *I have met someone who* [sic] *I really like. . . . Brad is the most wonderful, thoughtful, sincere, loveable, sensitive, cute person I've ever met. . . . He's so wonderful, I'm positive you'll be hearing about him for a long time to come.*

Supernatural psychic? Probably not. Despite my apparent gift for prophesy at age fourteen, I had no idea what "a long time to come" meant. One week was an *eternity* for me. I could not have predicted that eight years later, Brad and I would vow to love, honor, and cherish each other, for better or worse, for richer or poorer, in sickness and in health, till death do us part. I had no idea that ten years after that first night, Brad and I would toss our law school graduation caps into the air—or that I would later ditch my successful but unfulfilling legal career in a late-blooming effort to become a rock star. And, especially inconceivable to me on that first, magical night in 1985, at the tender age of fourteen, was the fact that, twenty-three years and two months later, I would clutch Brad for dear life, sobbing into his arms, having heard the doctor say "breast cancer" and "aggressive" and "chemotherapy." No, I didn't know any of those things on that first night. All I knew then, deep in my bones, was that I loved that boy.

Chapter 2

I sat trembling on the couch as I waited for Brad's arrival. His voice had flipped into commando mode when he'd said he was on his way. Why wasn't he here yet? I was starting to feel numb.

Call Dad, I thought. *I need to call Dad.*

I dialed Dad's cell phone.

"Dad," I began. I sounded pretty calm, actually. "Dad, it's . . . *c-c-can* . . ." I couldn't finish the word. I howled into the phone.

But Dad knew exactly what I was saying. "Oh, honey," he soothed. "I'm coming right now."

I told Dad not to come, that Brad would be home soon enough. But Dad knew his office was ten minutes closer than Brad's to my house, and he ignored me. Fifteen minutes later, I opened my front door and gratefully melted into his open arms. Later, he told me he'd had a horrible premonition a few nights earlier when I'd casually mentioned the biopsy; he'd had a feeling this was coming.

Fifteen minutes later, when Brad finally lurched through the front door and loped across the family room, scooping me up into his arms like a rag doll, I melted into his embrace. *Brad.*

How the hell did I get here?

Only two weeks before, a mere week before the biopsy, I'd signed a contract with a London-based record label for release of my music. At the ripe old age of thirty-seven! It was a dream come true, particularly since I'd spent the better part of the prior decade kicking someone's ass or having my ass kicked in courtrooms on a daily basis.

I hadn't mentioned The Lump or the biopsy to my new record label because I hadn't thought there was any chance I'd have a problem. Like Scarlett O'Hara—"fiddle dee dee!"—I didn't want to think about it. I had bigger fish to fry—like my imminent trip overseas to shoot a music video.

The record label had lined up a top-notch director with impressive credits: Paul McCartney! Lenny Kravitz! Annie Lennox! When John from the record label in London had talked about the "storyboard" for the video and "securing locations," I'd covered the telephone receiver with my hand to muffle my amateurish squeals of excitement.

"Act like ya been there before," Brad had coached me for years, usually after I'd spazzed out, yet again, in response to some trivial accomplishment.

But nonchalance just wasn't my strong suit.

And so, one week earlier, as we had driven to the hospital to biopsy the pea-size lump in my left breast, I hadn't been even a little bit concerned.

I'm not gonna get cancer just as my dreams are within grasp, I had thought. *Real life isn't a predictable Hollywood movie.*

And, anyway, bad things didn't happen to me.

Or so I had thought then.

Of course, later, I learned differently. Months later, after chemo had ravaged my hairless body, after I'd been reduced to frantically checking my fingernails each morning to see if they'd curled up and off during the night, after searing pain in my head and bones had caused me to cry out in a voice I did not recognize, I learned that, oh yes, bad things really did happen to me. But in the beginning, when scary words like "cancer" and "chemotherapy" had not yet attached themselves to my body in any tangible way, had not yet implanted their fish hooks in my flesh, I simply continued to float, uninterrupted, through the Hall of Scary Words like the Pollyanna I'd always been, those mean words bouncing off me like darts from a Nerf gun.

But Brad, unlike me, understood the gravity of the situation right from the start. During the biopsy procedure a few days before that stunning phone call from the surgeon, poor Brad sat anxiously in the waiting room for hours, all by himself, wringing his hands with worry and dread, as I drifted carelessly through the ether under general anesthesia.

According to Brad, when the surgeon finally emerged from the operating room, still dressed in green scrubs, the expression on his face made Brad's stomach drop.

"What is it?" Brad asked when the surgeon approached.

But the surgeon was noncommittal. "I don't know what that was. I've sent it to the lab for analysis."

Brad dusted off every trick in his long-abandoned lawyer bag, trying to pry a definitive answer from the surgeon. "Have you ever seen anything like it before? Was there anything about it that caused you concern? If you had to assign a percentage chance . . . "

But the doctor refused to elaborate.

And now, here we were, just a few days after that biopsy, driving to the surgeon's office in a haze of numbness, our worst fears realized, steeling ourselves to talk about my treatment options for . . . *cancer?* Brad drove the car, his white knuckles gripping the steering wheel as if we might veer uncontrollably off the road at any moment, while I blathered on and on in a state of shock, clinging desperately to my Teflon-coated reality.

"I'm going to be like Sheryl Crow," I proclaimed. "I'll have radiation, which will suck, but then I'll be cancer-free." And then, out of nowhere, I declared in a defiant tone, "You know I'm quitting the law, right?" I was daring him to contradict me. "I'm quitting the law," I said again for emphasis.

How could he possibly argue with me this time?

"Yes, baby," Brad said. "You just be a mommy now. You do whatever you want to do."

Even through my fog, I registered massive relief at his concession, the first of its kind after years of exhausting arguments on the topic. "I wanna quit law," I'd groaned (or whined, or yelled) through the years, to which Brad had always retorted, "Suck it up," or "We can't afford for you to quit," or "Stop being a wuss."

And now—how about that!—all it took was a little cancer diagnosis, and victory was all mine! *You do whatever you want to do,* he'd said!

I could finally kiss my law career goodbye!

Wow, I thought, snickering to myself, *Brad is gonna be annoyed with himself for backing down when we get to the surgeon's office and he confirms I have cancer lite.*

I returned to my blathering: "Radiation will suck," I continued, "but I'm going to be just fine. Just a bump in the road."

By the time Brad and I reached the surgeon's office, we had pulled ourselves together pretty well. We could handle this. I would be just like Sheryl Crow.

The surgeon informed us that it appeared we had caught the cancer early on.

See, just like Sheryl Crow.

The lump was very small, he said. So small, in fact, it was a medical marvel that I had been able to feel it at all. In a second surgery, he said, he'd remove more breast tissue and determine if the cancer had spread outside the breast and into the lymph nodes. If not, good! If yes . . . bad.

I just knew, without a doubt, there was no chance of a yes. It was simply out of the question.

"Do I need chemotherapy?" I wanted to know. This was his cue to pooh-pooh my question and tell me I was overreacting, to say I needn't worry, because, lucky for me, I had cancer lite.

But he didn't. "It's my guess you won't need chemotherapy,

Laura. But you'll need to talk to an oncologist about the specifics of your treatment plan."

All I heard him say was, "You won't need chemotherapy." Whatever else he said, if anything, sounded like popcorn in a microwave. *Pop, pop, pop.*

When I got home from visiting the surgeon, I called my office to talk to my law partner, Pete. For the past year, I'd been working in a small firm with Pete and another lawyer, old friends of mine from law school. Both guys, fathers themselves, genuinely supported my part-time schedule, knowing it afforded me irreplaceable time with my little girls. If ever I was going to enjoy being a lawyer, then working with these two sweethearts would have been the time. But even among such wonderful law partners, I still felt like a square peg in a round hole.

Over the past year in particular, my chosen career had turned me inside out with anxiety and insomnia. My biggest client, a loud-mouthed real estate developer named Frank, had been sued for millions of dollars by multiple investors in a new office complex, who claimed that Frank and his partners had bilked them out of profits on the deal. The lawsuits were threatening to run Frank out of business and into personal bankruptcy, too. On top of that, a few weeks earlier, as I'd defended Frank in this high-stakes contract dispute, he had been criminally indicted for allegedly defrauding investors in the same deal (which he vehemently insisted was a railroad job, and I actually believed him), his high-maintenance wife of fifteen years had filed for divorce, and, just to cap off the death-spiral trifecta, audited by the IRS.

I wasn't qualified or interested in defending Frank in criminal, divorce, and tax proceedings; I was a civil litigator. So he hired an army of legal specialists to fight his battles in each of his many lawsuits, the perfect storm of which would have sent a lesser man leaping off the nearest bridge. And now Frank's army of attorneys, coordinated by me, was fighting tooth and nail to preserve any shred of his life. Frank, understandably, called me multiple times per day in a state of utter panic, wanting to know his legal team's latest efforts. Every time I looked down at my phone, there was another voicemail from Frank, usually calling to inform me of yet another catastrophic turn in his life. I didn't know how this guy had avoided a heart attack up to this point; I felt like I was going to have one on his behalf, and it wasn't even my own life that was imploding so spectacularly.

"Frank," I told him during his fifth call of that particular day, "you've gotta stop calling me so much. Every time you call, it costs you money. Just think *cha-ching, cha-ching, cha-ching* every time you dial my number. I'm your lawyer, not your best friend."

Even under these horrendous circumstances, Frank still managed to laugh. He loved it when I straight-talked him. "But you're my best friend, Laura," he responded, his voice earnest. "I don't mind having to pay to talk to you."

Oh, geez. I'd become this guy's security blanket amid the biggest shitstorm of his life. I understood his desperation, but I didn't like being a paid hand-holder. "Frank, that's gross," I said matter-of-factly. "I can't be your woobie. You're a grown-ass man."

"But, Laura, you're all I have left."

My stomach seized. Indeed, my stomach had been in a permanent state of seizure for quite some time. I didn't want to see this guy go down. I actually liked him, quirky as he was. I thought my teeth were going to fall out of my head from the stress. In fact, I'd started having stress dreams involving teeth—crumbling teeth, shattered teeth, falling-out teeth. And, even worse, my lifelong problem with night terrors—nightmares on steroids, during which the sleeper screams or even runs around with his or her eyes open—was at a fever pitch. Many nights, I shrieked in terror as I witnessed imaginary home invaders, rats crawling all over the floor, or phantom figures jumping out of paintings in my sleep. I was losing my mind . . . and nearly causing Brad nightly cardiac arrest, too.

And now, on this particular day, when my own life had been hijacked to hell, there was no question that my days of fighting anyone's battles but my own were over.

I didn't mince words. "I have cancer," I told my law partner, Pete. "I'm not coming back to work."

Pete was compassionate, as was usual for him. "Laura, take as much time as you need. Your job is here for you when you're ready."

"Thanks, Pete. But no," I responded without hesitation. "I'm never coming back." I'd be damned if I was going to give up my cancer hall pass, my one-way ticket to freedom.

The next week was a whirlwind of MRIs, blood tests, and doctor's appointments in preparation for surgery. At each appointment, Brad was by my side, holding my hand or telling the technician to use a butterfly needle to draw blood because my veins are small. Brad never left my side. Literally. Every few minutes, he reached out to touch me—my face, my hair, my arm. At night, in bed together, we clutched each other in desperation and we cried. In fact, Brad cried more in that one week than he'd cried in the twenty-three years I'd known him.

"This wasn't in the script," he whispered over and over, tears streaming down his face. "This isn't how our story goes."

It killed me to watch Brad suffer like this—though, in truth, his passionate tears made me feel loved and appreciated like never before. And, yes, with each passing day, fear was tightening its stranglehold on me, too, as reality began sinking in and those Scary Words began embedding their insidious fish hooks deep in my flesh. But mostly, though I didn't dare say it out loud to anyone, I felt one overwhelming emotion above all others: relief. I'd finally found my golden ticket to freedom. And, by God, I wasn't going to waste it.

Chapter 3

A month after I'd first met Brad on that fateful night under the stars, my fifteenth birthday was fast approaching, in October 1985, and I was becoming increasingly anxious about having lied to him about my age during the past glorious weeks of our googly-eyed infatuation.

Maybe it won't come up, I thought. *Maybe he's forgotten what I said.*

But about a week before my fifteenth birthday, Brad asked, "Aren't you excited to get your driver's license?"

The jig was up—unless I could somehow fake getting my driver's license. I mulled that over for a moment. That would involve an elaborate web of lies, not to mention some illegal driving on my part. No, I couldn't pull that off.

There was no way out. I had to come clean.

"I'm actually turning *fifteen,* not sixteen," I confessed, wincing. "I lied."

I waited for Brad to tell me that my real age, or perhaps my initial deception, was a deal breaker. But, instead, he laughed and called himself a cradle robber. "What difference does it make?" he finally said. "Laura, you're such a knucklehead."

And that was that. The boy loved me.

When prom time arrived for Brad, who was a year ahead of me in school, I shrieked at the sound of his car in the driveway. With one last mirror check—yes, my silver dress was red-carpet ready and my hair and makeup were sheer perfection—I ran to the front door to greet him with a kiss.

"You look beautiful, Buddy," Brad said, as he slipped a corsage on my wrist.

He was right. I did.

At the raging party we attended before our dinner reservation, I took great care to dab the corners of my mouth with a cloth napkin after I'd gulped down a large cup of sweet-tasting, yellow-colored punch.

"Slow down, Buddy," Brad warned. "That punch has, like, four different liquors in it."

I smiled at him. I was fine.

An hour later, as Brad and I sat with three other couples at an elegant restaurant, I struggled to keep my head upright.

Does my head weigh thirty pounds? I wondered. It kept dipping down, as if I were a drowsy truck driver, and then I'd quickly whip it back up. I couldn't follow the conversations around me; all my energy was focused on keeping my head perpendicular to the table.

Suddenly, there was a burst of laughter from the group. I swung my head up and looked around, trying to see what was so funny. But I didn't notice anything.

"What?" I asked innocently.

Brad reached over to me and picked something out of my (perfectly coiffed) hair.

"You've got lettuce in your hair."

Apparently, that last head dip had collided most indelicately with my Caesar salad.

When college came a-calling for Brad, I still had my senior year to go, and I was worried.

"What if you meet someone else in college?" I asked anxiously as we sat, hand in hand, on a low beach wall, watching the setting sun merge with the shimmering ocean.

But Brad had decided to stay in town for college, and he was confident we'd survive. "Don't worry, Buddy," he assured me. "We'll be fine."

Out of nowhere, I felt an electric current zing right through my body. I'd never felt anything like it before. It was almost . . . supernatural.

"Oh my God," I gasped. I looked at Brad. "Do you feel that?"

His face registered shock, too. "Yes. I feel it."

We continued holding hands, this strange energy coursing between us. I looked around. Nothing seemed out of the ordinary for anyone else on the crowded beach. I looked at our hands. They looked completely normal.

"This is really weird," Brad whispered.

I started to cry, feeling overwhelmed with this indescribable electricity. Brad didn't ask me why I was crying. He could feel it, too.

After a few minutes, when the electric current had faded, Brad and I got up from our perch on the beach wall and made our way down the boardwalk, the whole time exchanging looks of disbelief.

There was no question from that day forward: We were meant to be together.

And yet when college came a-calling for me a year later, I could not escape the pull of my lifelong destiny to become the next Judy Garland. My destiny was bigger than me—bigger than Brad and me.

And I knew I needed to go to Hollywood, by way of the theater school at UCLA, to make it happen. And so Brad, the boy I loved so much, drove me to college to settle me into my dorm room.

It was my first giant step toward Judy-dom.

My heart had belonged to Judy Garland, the Most Beautiful Girl in the World, since I could remember. *Judy, Judy, Judy.* My Favorite Movie in the Whole World was *The Wizard of Oz.* I languished in eager anticipation of the movie's airing on television, as it did once a year around Easter time.

When the day I'd been waiting for finally arrived, Mom and Dad surprised me with the news that they were taking my older sister, Sharon, and me out to see a movie called *Rocky.* Sharon was thrilled, but I was beside myself with grief.

"*The Wizard of Oz* is on tonight!" I wailed, pulling at my hair.

Sharon rolled her eyes. "You can see it next year."

But I was adamant. I could not, *would not,* miss my beloved Dorothy and Toto. It was out of the question. *It would kill me!*

Mom and Dad had not intended to shatter their little girl's hopes and dreams; they'd just been in the mood for a movie. They lined up a baby sitter—Belinda, a heavy set teenager from down the street, whose jaw had been wired shut as part of her weight-loss plan—and off they went with a gloating Sharon to see *Rocky*.

Good riddance.

I sat, glued to the small TV in the family room, mouthing every line and singing along to every song. When Glinda asked Dorothy, "Are you a good witch or a bad witch?" I answered, in perfect mimicry of Dorothy's tone and inflection, "I'm not a witch at all!" My "lions and tigers and bears, oh my!" was a dead ringer for Dorothy's, too. In a film biography about Judy's life, I thought, I was a shoo-in to portray her as a child.

When my family returned home from seeing *Rocky*, Sharon could not stop yammering about the movie. She told me Rocky had spent a lot of time punching hanging meat. "And when he finally finished," she said, "he knew he was ready to fight Apollo Creed." She just couldn't stop flaunting her expertise on all things *Rocky*. She continued, looking smug, "Apollo was the champ, you know." Of course she knew I didn't know.

My interest was piqued. "Did Rocky win the fight?"

Another eye roll. "No. He *lost*." Sharon was exasperated. "*That was the whole point.*"

"He *lost*?!" *Well, that's just stupid.*

But Sharon told me it was so much better that he had lost. And, she said, I was a real dummy to miss having seen *Rocky* just so I could see a movie that would be on TV again next year. I didn't regret my decision, though, not even for a moment. Sharon could keep her stupid *Rocky*. I had my Dorothy.

That night, I was jolted awake from a horrible nightmare about the green-faced Wicked Witch of the West. She had locked me in her tower with the large hourglass, and the sands of time were rushing unabated toward the bottom. She cackled wickedly (of course) and called me "my pretty!"

I went into my parents' bedroom, frightened and crying, and woke them up.

"I had a nightmare, Mommy!"

Mom's thick hair was rumpled.

She retrieved something out of her dresser drawer, and then she led me back into my bed.

"Take this, lamby," she instructed. It was a tiny red satin pillow, maybe a sachet from her underwear drawer. She placed it in my hand. "This is a magic pillow. You can't have a nightmare if this is under your pillow." She smoothed my hair away from my face and kissed me on the forehead. "Now go back to sleep."

I rolled onto my side, feeling relieved and protected by my magic pillow, my new woobie. Nightmare-free sleep descended upon me. The sands of the hourglass were, thankfully, gone.

And now, thirteen years later, Brad and I sat in traffic, slowly making our way to the promised land of UCLA, the gateway to Judy-dom. I was taking control of my destiny, taking a giant leap toward the person I was meant to be!

So why, oh why, did it feel like my heart was being ripped out of my chest?

Chapter 4

"You're so smart, Buddy," Brad said, as we stood outside my dorm building at UCLA. "You're gonna do great." But his face was pained.

After one last hug, Brad climbed into his car to leave, blinking back tears. As he shut his car door, our eyes met and his mouth distorted. With an attempt at a smile and a little wave, he drove away, just as tears started streaming down his chiseled cheeks.

I sobbed under the shade of a nearby eucalyptus tree for an hour, and then finally made my way into my dorm room to meet my new roommates. My dorm "room" was actually a suite: two bedrooms, one tiny bathroom, and a small sitting area. In my bedroom, my two roommates were Kelly, a lily-white freshman majoring in engineering, and Naimah, an African American senior from Queens, New York. In the other bedroom, all three girls were of Asian descent: Marie had a wild mane of black hair and drove a Yamaha motorcycle, Erica was a girl-next-door type (literally, in this instance), and the last girl, my fifth roommate in the suite (whose name I cannot remember), was attached at the hip to her nebbish boyfriend, whom I did not particularly like. If the boyfriend had any charisma or social skills whatsoever, he did not reveal them to me.

After initial introductions and small talk, several of Naimah's friends came over with some beer, enough for all of us. After an hour or two, someone suggested we go swimming. This was a fab-u-lous idea, we all agreed, but, alas, the nearby university pool was closed for the night. But since it was hot and muggy, and by this time we were drunk, we didn't let a small thing like a locked fence change our plans.

Naimah's friend was a whiz at opening locked fences, it turned out, and in no time the group was cannonballing and chicken-fighting in the (closed) campus pool. But our boisterousness apparently alerted the cops, and soon Officer Bob was shining his flashlight into our stunned faces. When he yelled, "Freeze!" (wasn't that overkill?), time stood still for a nanosecond . . . until we hopped out of the pool and scattered like cockroaches after a kitchen light has been turned on.

I saw Naimah run into the dark, grassy field just west of the pool, and I followed her like a drunk driver tracking taillights. Clad in only our dripping-wet bikinis, Naimah and I played an enthusiastic game of follow-the-leader: She scaled a tall chain-link fence, and I followed. She jumped down to the sidewalk on the other side of the fence, and so did I. She ran for about a mile, straight to our dorm building, up the stairs, down the hall, and into our room. And I shadowed her.

Finally, Naimah and I were standing inside our dorm room,

leaning against the door, breathless, panting, and sweating through our soaking-wet bikinis. Only then did Naimah's eyes lock onto me— it was as if she were seeing me for the first time.

"Laura!" Naimah exclaimed in total surprise. "I had no idea that was *you* back there. I didn't know you had it in you." She was laughing. "Girl, you're all right."

I was beaming.

I didn't mention to Naimah that my lawlessness had been a singular fluke, or that, despite appearances, I really didn't have "it" in me at all. Wasn't college the perfect opportunity to reinvent myself?

I was now officially a badass.

Kelly and Erica, we later found out, had not run like fugitives from the law, like the rest of the group. Like proper law-abiding citizens, they had stood still when Officer Bob commanded them to "freeze!" But even though he had questioned them at the scene for almost half an hour, the girls had not ratted us out, much to our relief. Thankfully, Officer Bob had shown them mercy and let them go with a stern warning to relay a message to the rest of us to turn ourselves in. We all laughed and laughed about that one.

"Let me just go get my pants so I can run down to the police station," Naimah joked.

"Wait for me," I added. "I want to put on some makeup for the mug shot."

I sounded cavalier, but in actuality, I was scared to death that Officer Bob had tracked Kelly and Erica back to the dorms and would, at any given moment, burst into the room with a SWAT team. *Welcome to UCLA!*

The next day, I walked down the main artery on campus, enthralled by the thousands and thousands of diverse students swarming past me—black, white, Asian, and Latino!—and I felt like a country mouse in the big city. After having attended a small school with a graduating class of sixty-one—only one of whom was black—I found it electrifying to be a part of something so big. So *global*.

I was also proud to be at a big school with a storied sports program. Coach Wooden! Bill Walton! Jackie Robinson! Arthur Ashe! They were my people now.

One day, as I strolled through campus, I saw our Bruins quarterback, Troy Aikman (who went on to win three Super Bowls for the Dallas Cowboys), leisurely eating a cup of frozen yogurt, which looked like a thimble in his big hands. I walked past him without saying a word, but I wanted to scream at the top of my lungs, "This is UCLA, folks!"

I took general education classes all over campus, like Detective Fiction (a class well attended by the football team, I noticed) and Women's Studies (which prompted me to curse Brad's invidious attempts to "muzzle" me). But mostly I took classes for my theater major in a separate, "artsy" part of campus known as North Campus, where students lay on the grass in the sculpture garden, reading scripts, or lounged on benches, commiserating about upcoming auditions. I felt bohemian just being around them. And again, I was proud to be part of something with an illustrious history. Francis Ford Coppola! Carol Burnett! Lloyd Bridges! Jim Morrison! My peeps!

After my first week of school, Dad called to check up on me.

"Tell me the name of a fellow theater student who'll be famous one day," he challenged.

I didn't hesitate: "That's easy, Dad: Jack Black."

"Well, that's an easy one to remember," Dad responded, sounding excited.

Back in the dorms, whenever I was around Naimah, I tried, to the best of my ability, to "act like I'd been there before," just as Brad had always coached me.

Me? Verging on excited hysteria at all times? No sirree!

Naimah had turned out to be the coolest person I'd ever met, and I didn't want to alienate her by revealing my true personality. She was so cool, in fact, she was dating the biggest basketball star at UCLA. Once, I came home to the suite to find her and her boyfriend lounging on our no-frills dorm couch with Mike Tyson. Yeah, *that* Mike Tyson—the famous heavyweight boxer who was, back then, still undefeated and terrifying. Naimah introduced me to "Mike" and let me "chill" with their party in our sitting room. (Ever since our complicit run-in with the law, I'd earned a standing invitation to "hang" with Naimah and her friends—that is, if I didn't talk too much.) I sat there, staring at Iron Mike Tyson, such an anomaly in my dorm room, and tried to look unimpressed and relaxed.

His hardscrabble youth was etched all over his face, even as he laughed and bantered with Naimah's boyfriend. His laugh was unexpectedly high-pitched. Good God, the man's hands were massive. Those hands could kill you with one punch, I'd read somewhere.

Other than squeaking out a chipmunklike "hello" when Naimah briefly introduced me, I didn't utter a word the entire night.

As the school year progressed, Naimah and I encountered a troubling situation: Roommate No. 5's boyfriend had slept over every single night for the past two months. Why was this a problem, you wonder, since it was in the adjacent bedroom in my suite? Well, how about *you* try sharing one bathroom the size of a broom closet with five other girls, and then add one bonus guy on top of that? I'm certain you'd agree in a flash that this was an intolerable situation. But we didn't want to create World War III. Our living quarters were close enough without our creating conflict between the roommates.

Naimah and I hatched our plan.

As luck would have it, Naimah worked in the UCLA admissions office, so she was able to swipe one sheet of official UCLA letterhead. And on that official UCLA letterhead, I weaved my magic, writing a letter that went a little something like this:

March 3, 1989

To the residents of Hitch Suites, Room D-6:
It has come to our attention that one of you has been permanently housing a nonresident in your suite. Please consult your Hitch Suites Student Manual, section A.6, which explicitly prohibits nonresidents from staying overnight in any university housing complex.
We do not know which of you has committed this infraction, and we do not wish to know. If we receive any further information that a nonresident is residing in your rooms at any time, then all residents of Hitch Suites, Room D-6, shall

*be evicted with no additional warning. In that event, no
refunds will be provided.*

Sincerely,
Director of Student Housing, UCLA

I then made six copies of this missive and placed a copy in each
roommate's student mailbox, including Naimah's and mine. In due
course that day, each girl collected her mail and was surprised to receive
the startling letter. Apparently, none of the girls had noticed that the
letter was not signed, nor that the "Director of Student Housing" did
not even identify him/herself. No one even remotely suspected that
Naimah and I were the fraudulent "codirectors of student housing."

When Naimah and I sauntered into our suite, holding our letters
in our hands with looks of feigned incredulity, we encountered sheer
pandemonium already in progress. Marie and Erica were shouting at
Roommate No. 5's boyfriend. Erica, who'd been nothing but mild-
mannered and sweet up until then, was shouting that Boyfriend had
to get out!

"I'm not getting kicked out of here for you!" Erica screeched, her
eyes bulging with panic. "My dad would *kill me!*"

I joined in the sentiment, but oh so calmly and rationally, saying,
"Yes, I agree. If I get kicked out of student housing, my parents will
be quite upset with me."

That should have been it, right? Boyfriend should have said, "Of
course, ladies. I'm sorry I've jeopardized your housing situation. You
will never see me again." And with a sweep of his cape, he should

have been gone. But no, that's not what this immature little prick did. Instead, with veins bulging in his neck and left temple, he told us in a high-pitched whine that we girls were being "selfish."

Well, I lost it. "Selfish?!" I thundered. "You want to know what's selfish? Selfish is a guy who forces himself onto five unwilling roommates in an overcrowded dorm room with one bathroom. Now, that's what I call selfish!"

I had said my piece. If Boyfriend had kept his mouth shut at that point, I would not have uttered another word about it. But when that jerk had the nerve to then call me a bitch, I felt a rage I'd never felt before course through my body. I hurled myself toward him with the intention of beating him to a pulp—an impulse I have never otherwise experienced in my entire life. Naimah physically held me back, or I believe I would have thrown a haymaker on that guy. Boyfriend and Roommate No. 5 then left in a flurry of expletives and tears, never to return again (except at some point to collect Roommate No. 5's personal effects while everyone else was at class).

Erica hugged me and thanked me for backing her up, never suspecting that I had manipulated her into doing my dirty work in the first place.

Naimah, my accomplice, turned to me, winked, and said, "Girl, you're all right."

Chapter 5

"Mommy has some bad stuff in her breast—in her booby," Brad told our girls, Sophie and Chloe, ages eight and six, respectively. I sat next to him on the bed, trying to look unconcerned and casual. He continued, "But the doctor's already gotten it out. Just to be sure, though, the doctor's going to take out some more of the bad stuff next week."

The girls were fine with this calm explanation, until Brad admitted that the "bad stuff" was called cancer. Apparently, Sophie had heard this word before in connection with the death of a classmate's aunt, and she started wailing. Chloe, who'd initially thought cancer was something like chicken pox, now started crying, too, not fully understanding, but alarmed by her sister's reaction.

"Could you *die?!*" Sophie shouted at me between hysterical sobs.

"Oh, no!" I almost scoffed. "No, no. Some people die from cancer, it's true. And that is very sad. But my doctor caught this very early on, and he says there is no way I'll die." I figured if I was wrong about that, we'd cross that bridge when we got there.

I don't want to leave my girls, I thought. *I want to see them graduate from high school. I want to see them get married. I want to hold my grandchildren in my arms.*

I had always presumed I would do all those things. I was *entitled* to do those things, wasn't I? And, oh, I didn't want to leave poor Brad to raise those little girls all by himself. Brad. The love of my life. I had always thought I'd grow old with him. I had diligently put money into my 401(k) based on that assumption.

And my music. Oh, God, my music. I had only *just* discovered what I could do. Who I really was. My dreams, just now within my grasp, were over. *My dreams are over. My dreams are over. My dreams are over. My life is over. I am a cancer patient.*

But on that night, as we sat on Sophie's four-poster bed as a family, I didn't say what I was actually thinking. Instead, with a beauty-pageant smile plastered to my face, I proclaimed, "Everything's gonna be just fine."

A week later, after the surgeon had removed more of my breast and five lymph nodes from my armpit, I was socked in the gut by yet another damned phone call.

"I'm sorry, Laura," the surgeon said. "Lab tests are showing that the cancer has, indeed, metastasized outside the breast, into the lymph nodes."

I was speechless. Going into surgery, I had been told that the chances of this happening were slim, and I had relied on the percentages. I had still continued to believe nothing truly horrible could ever happen to me.

"This is a surprise," the surgeon continued. "With such a small lump, we had not expected the cancer to have spread. But that's the one thing you can count on with cancer: It's unpredictable."

Things had just gone from bad to worse. *I'm not gonna be like Sheryl Crow,* I realized, tears springing to my eyes. *This is not the way this was supposed to go.* I was starting to dislike talking to this guy.

"Thanks, Doc," I said when I finally managed a voice. "At least I know what I'm up against." I wanted to get off the phone and collect my thoughts. "So, I'll just make an appointment with the oncologist?" I was trying to wrap things up.

"Uh . . . there's more . . . "

Is this guy fucking kidding me? I waited. What more could there be?

The surgeon paused and cleared his throat. "Further analysis of the cells has revealed an extremely aggressive cancer. The cancer cells are multiplying at a very rapid rate. Really unusual."

I actually started to laugh. *Holy crap.*

A panic was seizing me.

Bad things were happening to me!

Hooks! Anchors! Spears! Invaders! I was being attacked!

"I'm so sorry, Laura."

Chapter 6

My best friend in the theater department, Amy (Amy Bo Bamy to me), had seen an ad in *Variety* seeking extras to play hippies in an upcoming movie about the Doors, by famed director Oliver Stone. A group of us donned flowing skirts, put flowers in our hair, and went to the cattle-call audition. I was a lock to get cast, I figured: I looked like I had just emerged from Woodstock.

As we hippie wannabes shuffled through a massive line, a casting director ordered everyone either "to the right" or "to the left." We didn't know what these designations meant. Did we want right or left? But when I got to the front of the line, the casting director said, "Go stand over there," indicating a man with a clipboard.

Hey, that's neither right nor left!

When I made my way over to the man with the clipboard, he took my picture with a Polaroid camera, scribbled something on a piece of paper, and then directed me to take his note to the costume trailer.

Costume trailer?!

When I got there, the costume lady told me I had been assigned to be a film student in a scene in which Jim Morrison (played by Val Kilmer) presented his student film at UCLA.

What? But I'm a hippie.

The costume designer fitted me in a '60s-ish miniskirt, button-down shirt, and loafers and told me to come back on the appointed day of filming.

Hy-per-vent-elation!

On the designated day, I arrived promptly for filming (repeatedly reminding myself it would be inappropriate to yell, "Action!" on set); got into costume, makeup, and hair (they brushed out my long, permed hair into an unattractive frizz-fest); and made my way to the crowded set. I was instructed where to sit in my scene, among a "classroom" of other students, and we then eagerly awaited the appearance of Oliver Stone and Val Kilmer. An hour later, Mr. Stone appeared on set, to our noisy applause. After explaining the scene and what he wanted us to do, he scanned the crowd and began singling out several people.

"You . . . you . . . you," he said, variously pointing. And then he looked right at me and said, "You."

My stomach lurched. *Me? Me!*

The small group—including *me!*—followed Mr. Stone to a corner of the set, at which time his assistant handed each of us a page from the screenplay—*the screenplay!*

"You're going to read for Girl One," the assistant told me.

No sooner had I glanced down at the page, trying to find the line attributed to Girl One, than Oliver Stone beckoned another girl and me over to him.

"Go," he said to the other girl, without prelude. She read the line, flustered. He then turned to me. "Go," he said. I read the line with gusto. He pointed to me. "You're it." Before I could speak, he walked away briskly.

And that, my friends, is how I snagged the illustrious and breakout role of Girl One in the epic, blockbuster, big-studio film *The Doors*.

When I sat back down in my designated seat on the set, the other extras now looked at me with awe and envy. *Who the hell is she? What's so special about her? I'm prettier than she is,* they thought. And, in all honesty, they were right. I could not account for Mr. Stone's selection of me. But I wasn't going to let him down.

As it turned out, Girl One was not intended to be a Grace Kelly type. She was not there to capture the leading man's eye or dance backwards in high heels with Fred Astaire. No, she was a symbol of the uptight establishment. Girl One wouldn't have understood true art if it had bitten her in the ass. Girl One was a total and complete bitch!

Here's the scene: Jim Morrison shows his disjointed and bizarre black-and-white student film to his UCLA film class. The camera pans to the student audience, showing various people reacting to the film—including one frizzy-haired young woman with oily skin. She makes an exaggerated look of disgust (subtlety, apparently, not being her specialty).

After Morrison's short film is over, the lights come up and the professor, played by Oliver Stone himself, says something like, "This is pretty shocking stuff, Mr. Morrison. Nazism and masturbation? Not sure what you were trying to do there." Then, motioning to the class, he asks, "What do you all think?"

A male student says, "It was better than a Warhol picture." The crowd erupts in agreement or disagreement—I'm not sure which.

And then (drum roll, please) . . . the frizzy-haired, shiny-faced girl says . . . (*ahem*—silence, please), "No, it wasn't. It was worse!"

At this point in the filming, Mr. Stone stopped and said, "Whoa! Girl One, that was the most poignant performance I have ever been honored and privileged to witness. Thank you for sharing your art— your *soul*—with us today." And then the entire room, including Val Kilmer, stood up and applauded for a full six minutes.

Okay, that last part didn't happen. But the frizzy-haired girl most certainly did utter her line with aplomb, and the room really did erupt, as instructed by Mr. Stone, with emotional reactions to her apparent inability to recognize true art.

Continuing the scene: The professor (Mr. Stone) turns to Jim Morrison (Val Kilmer) and says (something like), "Okay, okay [*responding to the outburst from the class*]. Mr. Morrison, what are your feelings on this?"

And Mr. Morrison/Val Kilmer, sitting at the front of the class on a little step, quietly says, "I quit." And then he walks out.

Scene!

You might be surprised to learn that it took over eight hours to shoot that little scene. An entire day! And I was paid by the hour, too! *And* I was treated to a fabulous lunch of chicken and rice, catered by craft services!

When I sat down at lunchtime to eat my scrumptious meal with my fellow extras, everyone wanted to hear the story of how on earth I had snagged the coveted part of Girl One. Of course I obliged, repeatedly—feeling like a special young lady, indeed.

At the end of the long, hot day (during which any makeup that had been applied to my oily face melted off), one of the crew pulled me aside to make sure he had the correct spelling of my name. After all, he said, he wanted to be sure it would be listed correctly in the credits. *The credits?!* Yes, the credits. As Girl One, he told me. It was too good to be true. Not only that, but this little speaking line would get me into the Screen Actors Guild, something countless aspiring actors aimed to accomplish. Heaven!

How would I ever be able to wait a full year for the movie to come out in theaters so I could see my name in lights? Waiting was going to be sheer agony!

What I needed was another exciting adventure to distract me as I awaited my destiny. As luck would have it, a few weeks later, Amy Bo Bamy and I were invited to appear as lowly extras in another scene in the movie, accompanied by our friend Marco Sanchez, a ridiculously good-looking guy of Cuban descent (who joked he was actually an Irishman named Marc O'Sanchez). The scene was being shot at the famed Whisky a Go Go, a music club in Hollywood where the Doors, along with other rock icons like Jimi Hendrix and Janis Joplin, had made rock 'n' roll history in the '60s. Unlike with my earlier classroom scene, there was no question this time around that I would be an uncredited extra, known (only to myself) as "the girl in the yellow-and-red-checkered minidress." But that was fine with me—I'd already secured my ticket to superstardom in the UCLA film school scene, so this additional chance to be on camera was just an unexpected bonus.

In the scene, the (pretend) Doors, led by Val Kilmer, who writhed around in tight leather pants that left nothing to the imagination, performed the song "The End," the Doors' lengthy, Oedipal song culminating in Jim Morrison's shouting that he wants to "fuck" his mother and "kill" his father, as the crowd, which included Amy, Marco, and me, tried to act like we'd never heard anything like this before.

For angles focusing on the crowd's reactions, in which only the lower half of Kilmer's body was visible in the frame, a body double wearing identical black leather pants came onstage to assume writhing duties. As we tried to look as if we were witnessing the most progressive rock performance we'd ever seen, the body double, who apparently had never seen footage of the real Jim Morrison in action, gracefully danced jetés and pirouettes across the stage.

In "the end" (just a little Doors humor for you), Marco, Amy, and I were treated to at least sixteen billion simulated performances of "The End" over the course of our sixteen hours at the Whisky (and an equal number of graceful pirouettes by Val Kilmer's dance double). And through it all, a fierce yearning bubbled and simmered inside my veins: I longed to join the ranks of Jim Morrison, Janis Joplin, Jimi Hendrix, and Val Kilmer—and, hell, even Val Kilmer's clownish double—front and center onstage at the Whisky a Go Go.

It was only a matter of time before my destiny would be fulfilled, I knew. Once the movie had premiered, probably in about a year, the world would be captivated by my groundbreaking performance as Girl

One, and my Hollywood career would be on the fast track. I simply had to exercise superhuman patience until that fateful day arrived.

When the movie finally came out, Brad and I practically sprinted to the theater. As the lights dimmed, he squeezed my hand and grinned at me with excited anticipation. We were on the edge of our seats.

We didn't have to wait too long for my big moment: The UCLA film school scene was one of the first in the movie.

Oh my God, there I was. There was my school bus–size, shiny face, framed by my massive mop of frizzy hair, reacting with cartoonish repulsion to Jim Morrison's student film—my over-the-top facial expression more reminiscent of a 1920s silent-film star encountering the Mummy than of the second coming of Meryl Streep. And then there I was *again,* in yet another extreme close-up shot, uttering my now famous line—"No, it wasn't. It was worse!"—with a cringe-inducing zeal smacking of Darla from *The Little Rascals.*

I should say that I was jubilant—two full-screen reaction shots *and* a speaking line!—but the truth is, I was just in shock at how unattractive and unnatural I looked on film. Did I really look like that? Had my performance really been that bad?

Hold it together, Laura, I thought. The Whisky a Go Go scene was still coming. Surely I hadn't screwed that up, too.

But when the Whisky scene appeared onscreen, there was nary a glimpse of "the girl in the yellow-and-red-checkered minidress." Not a glimpse!

I was crestfallen.

The ending credits began to roll. *My greatest glory still awaits me,*

I realized. It was time to behold my name in lights in a big-budget studio film. I was Girl One, damn it, and no one could ever take that away from me, crappy performance and all.

Brad squeezed my hand and we scanned the torturously long list of names scrolling down the screen, our anticipatory excitement threatening to spout like a geyser. Okay, there were the lead actors' names: Val Kilmer, Meg Ryan, Kyle MacLachlan . . . yes, yes. Now there was someone credited as "Indian in Desert."

The names continued to scroll. "Bouncer." "Bartender."

We scanned . . . and scanned . . . and scanned. And scanned. Where was I? There was "Girl in Car." Not quite.

Finally, yes, here was some guy credited as "UCLA Student." But where was my name? Shouldn't my name appear next to his?

Now the credits had moved on to technical contributors: make-up, sound, casting director, transportation. *Transportation?*

Where the hell was I?

And then the lights came up. Movie over. My name had not been listed.

Brad and I sat silently in our seats for a long moment as streams of moviegoers shuffled past us in the aisles.

"I hated it," I finally mumbled after several minutes, my gaze still directed at the now blank movie screen in the empty theater.

Brad, who knew me so well, hugged me without saying a word.

I haven't seen the movie since.

Chapter 7

As much as my doctor's initially uttering the word "cancer" cut me at the knees, the word "aggressive" as a modifier for "cancer" was a sucker punch to the jaw. And then, two days after I heard that my "aggressive cancer" had spread outside my breast—much to the surprise of my doctor—the damned surgeon called yet again.

By this time, I hated the sound of that son of a bitch's voice. "Hey, Doc," I greeted him wearily, resigned to the fact that he was undoubtedly calling with more bad news. "What's new?"

"Laura, we've done further lab testing." *Enough with the lab testing already!* "Your cancer cells are unusual; they've tested negative for three receptors typically found on cancer cells." *What the hell does that mean?* "In recent years," the surgeon continued, sounding professorial, "we've made great strides in treatment by targeting these receptors.

It's rare to find cancer cells without even one of them." *Did he just say the word "rare"?* Another sucker punch.

I paused, waiting for more. But apparently he was finished. "What does this mean for my treatment?" I asked mechanically. No tears came. Just numbness. Resignation. Those Scary Words had now anchored their hooks deep inside my chest cavity, in my organs, in my heart. It was too much to defend against, too much to rise above.

"Well," he said, "it would be best for an oncologist to explain the recommended treatment for this particular type of breast cancer."

Well, thanks a whole hell of a lot.

Was I imagining all of this? Or, even worse, had I manifested a disaster of this proportion as a desperate ploy for attention?

When I was seven or eight, my sister, Sharon, went to the hospital overnight to get her tonsils removed. I was so pea green with envy about all the presents and attention she got—she even got to eat ice cream for dinner!—that I tried to break my own leg, leaping off the three-foot retaining wall in front of our house over and over. But, alas, I didn't have the courage to land awkwardly, and my damned stick legs never broke. Was all of this just another pathetic attempt to garner attention and presents?

After the "you've got a rare and aggressive form of cancer" phone call from the surgeon, Brad disappeared immediately into his study to gather information online. Several hours later, he emerged to tell me he had figured out my diagnosis: I had something called "triple negative breast cancer." Doctors had discovered its existence only about five years ago, he said.

"Because it's really aggressive and shows up quickly," Brad explained (having obtained his MD online in a matter of hours), "it's typically seen in younger women, like you." He stared at me expectantly, but I didn't say anything. "Only about ten percent of breast cancers are triple negative," Brad continued, astonishing me with his infinite expertise. Really, forget real estate brokerage; he should have been saving the world with his oncology. "And of that ten percent, the disease mostly strikes African American women. Only a small percentage of triple-negative girls fit your profile."

"So, I'm the minority profile among patients with a rare kind of cancer?" I summarized. I was always striving to be unique, but this was ridiculous.

Brad tried to lighten the mood with humor. "Why do you have to be top two percent in everything you do?"

I appreciated his attempt to add levity to the situation, especially given how emotional we'd both been over the past week, but I wasn't about to take his word for my diagnosis, thank you very much. "I'll wait for an actual doctor to tell me what I have," I told him. I was snippy. "It might not be this triple-negative thing."

"It *is* triple negative," Brad persisted.

"I'll just wait to hear what the oncologist says." Now I was pissy. "I'm not going to play armchair oncologist based on information from the Internet."

Over the next few days, Brad and I consulted three different oncologists, seeking second and third opinions. And guess what? They all said the same thing.

Diagnosis: triple negative breast cancer.

Brad was right. *Damn.*

Treatment: (1) eight chemotherapy infusions, administered every two weeks, and after those, (2) radiation therapy, administered five days a week for about seven weeks.

Double damn. I hated it when Brad was right. Especially about this.

Chapter 8

At the end of my first year at UCLA, I moved into an off-campus apartment with a fellow theater major named Holly. I commuted to and from my new apartment on a lawn mower–size scooter, wearing a black, Darth Vader–style helmet that was bigger than the scooter itself. One day, an old lady in a sedan left-turned in front of me as I was riding my scooter to class, causing my massive helmet (with my head inside) to crash right through her driver's side window.

As I lay on the asphalt, dazed and incredulous among the sprays of glass all over the street, I could see looky-loos gawking at me from their apartment balconies.

They're looking at me, I mused. *I'm the accident.*

Despite a sirens-blaring ambulance ride to the hospital and a few bruises and scratches, I was perfectly fine, though. Better than fine, actually—within a few days, I picked up a check for about $6,000 in a legal settlement from the old lady's insurance company. I was living large. Even after a collision, I still came out ahead. Nothing bad ever happened to me.

Six thousand dollars might as well have been $6 million to a nineteen-year-old, and it was burning a hole in my pocket. On a weekend visit home to San Diego, Brad and I wandered aimlessly into a pet store, saw a puppy mill–bred, black-and-white Boston terrier with bug eyes and bat ears, and purchased him on the spot. No planning, no forethought; we just thought he was so ugly, he was cute. We named him Buster—actually, Buster Francis Martín Hoffman. ("Roppé" later became affixed to the end of that, after Brad and I tied the knot.)

Buster had a smashed-in face only a mother could love. When I was walking him along a busy street, a car pulled over alongside me and the driver yelled out, "Is that a *pig!?*" And, in addition to his being ugly-cute, we came to find out the damned dog was a lunatic. He barked and attacked like a velociraptor when we tried to leave the house. And, though typically affectionate, he might, without warning, fly into an uncontainable rage toward any creature he viewed as either vulnerable (like a golden retriever puppy) or a threat (like a full-grown Rottweiler). He was disgusting, too: He farted and snorted, and tunneled his way under our covers to the foot of the bed, then came out gasping for air when he could no longer breathe (due to either the suffocating blankets or the fumes his nonstop farting created).

I'd had no luck training Buster, so I figured maybe a superhero doggie trainer could whip him into shape. Of course, this being L.A., I had struck up an acquaintance with an Irish "dog trainer to the stars," who looked just like Bono and frequented the dog park across the street. For a hefty sum paid up front (again, I guess that settlement money was burning a hole in my pocket), the trainer agreed to provide twelve weekly one-on-one training sessions.

Each week I took Buster to this Irish dog trainer, and he dragged and pulled Buster around the park on a leash as if Buster were a wet beach towel on a rope. "Heel!" Bono the Irish dog trainer commanded. "Heel, Buster! Heel! Heel! Heel! *Heel!*"

It didn't seem like Buster was heeling, but I figured the guy knew what he was doing. Six weeks into training, though, Bono came to me and said apologetically, in his sweet Lucky Charms lilt, "Please don't tell anyone about this. I've got a reputation to maintain, I do *(dewe)*. But your dog would sooner die *(diye)* than mind me." And then he unceremoniously placed a full refund in my hand.

The refund was a nice chunk of change, but, thanks to my recent spending spree, it was just a drop in the bucket. I needed money.

I got a job working as a valet parker at Hollywood parties, parking the Porsches, Bentleys, and Lamborghinis of the stars. George Burns (so old)! Sidney Poitier (so elegant)! There I was, nineteen years old, dressed in my red valet jacket, black slacks, and black sneakers, parking cars worth more than I would earn in my lifetime. I couldn't imagine a better job.

At one particularly raging Hollywood party, Robert Downey Jr., one of my all-time favorites, emerged and nonchalantly handed me his valet ticket.

"Right away!" I chirped, and flew to the nearby lot to find his car, which turned out to be a stunning black Porsche. I had just recently been drooling over Robert Downey Jr. in *Less Than Zero,* and now I was sitting in the driver's seat of his car. *My hands are touching where his hands touch,* I thought, as I gripped his steering wheel. *My butt is touching the exact spot where his butt touches.* I smiled. There was only one degree of separation between our butts' touching each other. I was in sheer ecstasy.

I wanted to savor this moment, memorize the scent of him lingering on his finely appointed leather bucket seats, but, alas, I had work to do. With a sigh, I turned the key in Robert Downey Jr.'s ignition and carefully made my way back to the party.

As I drove the car toward the front of the club, there he was, standing on the curb, chatting with his pretty date.

Lucky girl, I thought about Robert's beautiful companion. And, my God, she really *was* beautiful.

I pulled the car up to the curb, and Robert came over to the driver's side door. Just as I reached out to open the door, Robert opened it for me with a dramatic flourish, as if I were a star arriving at a movie premiere.

Robert, in the role of Valet Parker, held out his hand to me, Young Starlet—and, with a broad smile, I slid my hand into his.

Warmth spread throughout my body as he pulled me out of his car and up to a standing position, close to him.

And then there I was—gushing, smiling, blushing, beaming— *standing face-to-face with Robert Downey Jr.* He kissed the top of my hand and said, "My lady." And then he twirled me and dropped me into an elegant dip, instantly transforming my red valet-parker jacket and black slacks into a feathery gown.

When I came back up, flushed and speechless, he bowed deeply and formally to me, to which I responded with something like, "*Grf.*"

Robert smiled his dazzling, warm smile and gestured to the small crowd on the curb for applause (which, of course, he received). He then handed me a $20 bill as a tip, got into his sparkling black Porsche (with that sparkling woman sitting right beside him), and sped away into the night, taking a tiny piece of my heart with him into eternity.

I stood for a long moment, watching Robert Downey Jr.'s red taillights speeding away.

Lucky girl, I thought again. But this time, that lucky girl was me.

Oh, how Robert Downey Jr.'s random act of kindness that night put a spring in my step! Of all the gin joints in all the towns in all the world, he had walked into mine. My goose bumps didn't subside for *weeks*.

And on top of that, the man was a great tipper! Twenty dollars was a helluva lotta clams for a young girl like me, particularly since *I* would have paid *him* one hundred times that amount to play Ginger Rogers to his Fred Astaire, just for that fleeting, fairytale moment.

But the truth was, although Robert's big tip was much appreciated, it was not unusual for me. I raked in the dough as a valet parker. For one thing, I was bubbly and vivacious and obviously having an epically good time. I was thrilled down to the tips of my toes every time I caught even a glimpse of a movie star. And I was giddy with excitement each time I got behind the wheel of a Lamborghini, Porsche, or Ferrari—if only to drive it to a parking garage one hundred yards away. I'm sure my benefactors got a kick out of my unabashed exuberance for valet parking.

But let's be honest: The real reason for my customers' largesse was that I was the only female parker in the entire company (not to mention the only English-speaking parker on any given team). It was like taking candy from a baby. Man, oh man, *I worked it!* I chatted and charmed and laughed and smiled. And I'm pretty sure I hair-flipped a time or two (or thirty) as well. Money just fell out of the sky and into my grateful hands like gum drops raining down in Candy Land.

At the end of each shift, my fellow valet parkers and I threw our tips into a common pool and then split everything equally. My first three or four shifts, I contributed fives, tens, and twenties to the collective pot, while the other poor saps put in dollar bills. It didn't take too long before I wised up and started bringing a wad of singles with me to the job. From that point on, I threw dummy tips into the pot after each shift, having furtively stuffed my bonanza of real tips into my bra.

Sadly, when the white-haired, fiftysomething-year-old manager of the valet parking company asked me to join him for a weekend trade show in Las Vegas—just him and me—it was time to quit the job, though I loved it so.

Still in need of some extra cash, I got a job at a Beverly Hills rare-coin store, even though I didn't know the first thing about coins. If a customer had a question about a particular coin, I'd smile politely and say, "Just a moment, please," and then I'd find the store owner, who slaved away (at who knows what) in an office in the back.

On my lunch breaks, I walked up and down Rodeo Drive, window shopping at the fancy stores and gawking at supernaturally beautiful women as they click-clacked past me in their stiletto heels and designer dresses. I was always, always, on the lookout for a movie star on a shopping spree, but to no avail.

And then one afternoon, the little bell over the front door jingled and in walked one of my all-time favorites, the regal and beautiful Anne Bancroft.

Anne Bancroft! Mrs. Robinson!

"Hello," Anne Bancroft greeted me. She handed me a gold coin. "Can you please tell me the value of this?"

That voice! I recognized that voice! I could hear it asking a young Dustin Hoffman, "Do you want me to seduce you?"

And that face! That gorgeous face, conveying earthiness and elegance all at once. This was a woman of *substance.*

I could not speak, I was so enthralled.

I nodded, smiled a goofy smile, and took the coin from her outstretched hand.

With my eyes glued to her iconic face, I turned to walk to the back of the store. I was so starstruck, however, that I smacked into the wall behind me, banging my forehead with a loud *thud.*

When I turned sheepishly back around, touching the already rising lump on my forehead, Anne Bancroft flashed me a loving, maternal smile.

I gratefully returned her smile, a bit embarrassed, and made my way gingerly to the back of the store.

"Anne Bancroft's out there!" I stage-whispered to the store owner, holding out the coin. "Mrs. Robinson!"

With a loud exhale, he leaped up from his desk, plucked the coin from my hand, and bustled away, murmuring, "Stay here!"

I stayed behind, as instructed, but I watched the festivities through a crack in his office door: Mrs. Robinson listened intently to the store owner's pontifications, her head cocked and her eyebrows questioning; Mrs. Robinson took the coin back with a polite "thank you"; Mrs. Robinson walked out of the store, apparently not satisfied with whatever the store owner had said.

And that's when it hit me: This was no coincidence. Anne Bancroft hadn't randomly wandered into my rare-coin store!

No, Anne Bancroft was a sign from the universe, an answer to my rain dance—a glimpse into my glorious future.

Anne Bancroft was a harbinger of my destiny.

Here's to you, Mrs. Robinson!

Chapter 9

It had finally sunk in: I had triple negative breast cancer. I was going to have to fight for my life. Like Debra Winger in *Terms of Endearment*. Except wait—she died in that movie. Scrap that.

Just a few weeks before, I'd *finally* resumed dancing and singing my way down the Yellow Brick Road toward Judy-dom—a *lawyer* had signed a midlife record deal?!—and now, after one disorienting phone call, I had been swept up by a flying monkey and secreted away in the Wicked Witch's tower, with nary a yellow brick in sight.

My brain wasn't functioning normally, and my body felt dragged down by fifty-pound weights. Just taking air into my lungs and then expelling it required a massive effort. Making a grilled cheese sandwich for Chloe was a Herculean feat.

I cried easily and often.

My face felt heavy. Numb. I was sinking, sinking, sinking into darkness.

And Brad wasn't faring any better.

Brad had never been a crier; I could remember only a handful of times I'd seen him cry in the twenty-three years I'd known him. And yet now he could not contain his despair. While I put on a brave face to watch a movie with the girls, Brad skulked off to our bedroom to cry in private, and then, when I could no longer maintain my stiff upper lip, we'd switch places. At night, after the girls had gone to sleep, we lay in bed together, relieved to be able to break down together in the privacy of our bedroom. Every night, we clutched each other like rock climbers clinging to a boulder.

The closest I'd ever come to feeling this way was when my beloved childhood dog, Darrow, died in his old age during my senior year of high school. Back when I was five, my parents came home from a weekend away with a black-and-white terrier mix from the pound. Almost hyperventilating with joy, I stormed outside, into the middle of the street, and shouted at the tippy-top of my lungs, "We got a puppy!"

At this, children swarmed out of neighboring houses and into our back yard, eventually huddling tightly around the main attraction. Amidst our shouting and cooing, that poor, overwhelmed puppy yakked, and then, on wobbly legs, teetered, with hardly a splash, right into the swimming pool. Like a superhero, Dad scooped the soggy ball of fur out of the water with our blue pool net and plopped him back onto the patio.

"What should we name him?" Dad asked later, when the commotion had died down.

"Lemon Drop," Sharon suggested.

"Fruity," I proffered.

But Dad, a Stanford-educated attorney and the man I loved most in the whole world, dismissed our suggestions with a wave of his hand. "We'll call him Darrow," he declared with full authority, "after the famous trial lawyer Clarence Darrow."

And thus Dad foretold, or perhaps even charted, my future.

When Darrow died as an old dog, I lovingly laid every single photo of him ever taken on my bed, creating a makeshift shrine, and then reclined facedown right on top of them, my heart disintegrating like plastic wrap in a microwave, my grief a bottomless well. For three days, I wailed my lungs out on top of those photos, not knowing how to climb out of my dark hole.

I'd adored Darrow's hangdog eyes and tear-sopping fur—and his pragmatic advice through the travails of my childhood had always been right on the money. No matter how much I had pestered him—trying repeatedly but in vain to perform the *Lady and the Tramp* spaghetti trick with him, or forcing him to emulate the closet scene from *E.T.* by peeking his head out of my stuffed-animal collection—he had offered unwavering and uncomplicated companionship.

On the third day of my grief at losing my little four-legged attorney, Brad came over, kissed my swollen eyelids, and said, "Baby, you've got to pull yourself together now." And so I did.

But this—this horrific diagnosis, this looming death sentence of mine—was exponentially more excruciating than losing my beloved Darrow, though I'd have jumped in front of a moving train for him.

And this time, Brad was in no condition to stitch up the gaping hole in my heart. He was falling apart, too. At night, as we lay in bed, clutching each other, he whispered, "I can't live without you" over and over, and tightened his grip on my body as if he could prevent me, by sheer force of will, from slipping away.

The thought that Brad could not survive without me—perhaps literally—terrified me, since, I figured, he might not have a choice in the matter. But that wasn't what I told him on those nights as we lay, just the two of us, holding each other in the dark.

"I'm gonna be fine," I reassured him, stroking his tear-stained cheeks. I was amazed at how calm and assured my voice sounded.

"Do you promise?" His voice was shaky.

"Yes, Buddy. I promise."

If that promise turned out to be a lie, I reasoned, and if survival just wasn't in the cards for me after all, Brad would simply have to forgive me.

Chapter 10

When we'd both graduated from college, Brad moved to L.A. to live with me while I pursued my big Hollywood dreams, even though he didn't fully understand them.

"You're so smart," he said. "You should be inventing the cure for cancer."

But I didn't want to invent the cure for cancer. I wanted to be a *star*.

We got an airy apartment that allowed pets, for Crazy Buster. Our next-door neighbor was a perpetually harried woman with six snorting pugs, and the guy upstairs had a loud (goddamned) bird. Brad got a job in the copy department of a law firm while he figured out his next move. And I, presumably, set out to "make it."

I managed to book an audition with a reputable talent agent in the Valley. A successful audition could be a life-changing opportunity. A theater friend of mine named Rob agreed to perform a dramatic scene with me, and we rehearsed and rehearsed. Finally, the big day arrived and we performed our scene for the agent in his Burbank office.

"Compelling," he complimented Rob first. "You're understated and believable."

And then he turned to me. "You're good," he said. "But . . . we've already got one of you."

Before I could ask him what "having one of me" meant, he elaborated: "We already represent Martha Plimpton."

What? I was the poor man's Martha Plimpton?

Surely, someone out there would be able to appreciate my special Laura-ness. I was unique! Unlike anyone else! I was not some shoddy Martha Plimpton mimeograph, thank you very much.

I got a head shot made, and I mailed it out to every reputable talent agent in the greater Los Angeles area. I'd show that guy!

And then, by God, I waited . . . and waited.

But I didn't get a single response to my head shot mailings.

"I think I'll go to law school," Brad declared eight weeks later, having long since abandoned all inquiries about the progress of my talent-agency mailing.

And I, the former star of *The Doors,* the girl once destined to become the next Judy Garland, the purveyor of a unique brand of Laura-ness not heretofore seen anywhere else in the world, shrugged my deflated shoulders and said, "Me, too."

So much for polishing my Oscar-acceptance speech.

Why the change of heart? Because the rubber had finally hit the road on an internal wrestling match I'd been waging my whole life: In one corner, there was my heart—my creativity and dreams—looking sort of like a headband-clad Ralph Macchio in the original *Karate Kid.* In the other corner, there was my head, looking surprisingly like Ralph Macchio's blond nemesis in that same movie, standing with a combative expression on his (its) face. *I'm superior to you,* my head taunted my heart. *I'm analytical, pragmatic, and far more respected by society . . . and by your family, too.* And with that, my head landed a roundhouse kick on my heart.

I'd been told from a young age by my family and teachers that I was off-the-charts smart, and I took their opinions in this regard to be unquestionable fact. If it was true that I was a brainiac, as the adults said, then I supposed I'd better not waste my big, fat brains on pursuits for dummies—even though most of the left brain–centered classes, like algebra and chemistry, were torturous. To do otherwise would be such a waste, and a disappointment to everyone, wouldn't it? And yet if I were to pursue others' projections of me to fruition, rather than what bubbled inside me like molten lava, how would I ever achieve Judy-dom? Over time, I reconciled the conflict this way: In addition to winning the Academy Award one day, I'd also invent the next Ziploc bags or achieve some other history-changing feat, too. That seemed like a fair solution.

With each passing year, I felt the strain of my inner conflict: Should I surrender to the allegedly analytical and conventional person others seemed to value in me, or let my freak flag fly and unabashedly pursue my name in lights?

On the first day of my senior year of high school, I sat in Mr. Brown's trigonometry class, a Cheshire cat–like grin across my face, smug about the fact that, unbeknownst to anyone else, I'd staged an illicit protest. I had been slated to take calculus that year, but instead I'd covertly signed up for trigonometry—one step *behind* the advanced algebra course I'd completed the year before.

I'd spent the last three years of high school studying myself into a stupor, and, by God, I was going to enjoy my senior year, especially now that Brad was embarking on a party-filled freshman year at the local university. Besides, I needed to free up more time for the one thing that had unlocked my soul more than anything else: singing. I had starred in every high school musical, and I'd reveled in every minute of every performance—except for the time when my shirt fell off in the middle of a performance, leaving me standing, aghast, at center stage in my Maidenform bra and the audience gasping, "Oh!" in unison. And so I had decided, at least for my senior year of high school, that it was high time for my heart to reign supreme.

As Mr. Brown drew a figure on the white board, the classroom door opened and the calculus teacher stormed into the room. The class looked up at him expectantly, full of dread. The calculus teacher surveyed the room, until his eyes fixed on me.

"You," he said, pointing. "You're supposed to be in calculus. Come with me."

Please! Don't hurt me. "I'm not taking calculus this year," I said meekly.

He paused, assessing me. "Tell that to Mrs. Beldam."

With all eyes staring at me, and a few scattered snickers, I excused myself and made my way to the assistant headmistress's office.

Mrs. Beldam was a stark woman who invoked terror in every student—even more so than the actual headmaster, who happened to be her husband. Even her smiles were chilling. Think Nurse Ratched in *One Flew Over the Cuckoo's Nest*. Or maybe, more aptly, the Wicked Witch of the West.

"You are supposed to take calculus this year, Laura," Mrs. Beldam said, her voice steely. It was petrifying to hear her utter my name. "Trigonometry is a step backwards for you," she continued. "This is most unlike you, Laura." Again, terror.

"I'm not . . . really . . . interested in taking calculus this year," I answered.

She let this information set in. Her expression was one of disappointment and disdain; apparently, I was not the scholar she had presumed.

"Do your parents know about this . . . my pretty?"

"Yes, they do."

Well, implicitly. When a kid barricades herself regularly in her room to study for hours on end, there's no need for parental pressure, is there?

"Is calculus a required course?" I asked, but I knew the answer. *You can't make me!*

"No," she answered with reluctance. She was pissed.

"Okay, well, then, I'll just stick with trigonometry."

And with that, I hurled a bucket of water at her face and then leaped back in horror as she started fizzling and melting into a puddle on her desk.

"Oh, what a world, what a world!" she howled amid the rising steam.

"May I go back to class?" I asked, sweetness personified.

She stared me down. "Go ahead." She shot daggers at me.

I skipped back to class, resisting the urge to whistle. I had stood my ground against a powerful, green-faced witch and had adhered to my principles—even if my newfound principles were laziness, sloth, and lack of ambition. I'd avoided evil calculus, ensured a glorious senior year with my college-freshman boyfriend, and paved the way for my continued pursuit of Judy-dom.

And then, at the end of the school year, I marched off, triumphantly raising Mrs. Beldam's broomstick into the sky, all the way to the theater school at UCLA.

Score one for the heart.

And yet only a few short years later, by the time of my college graduation, my head had stormed back and waged a come-from-behind victory, relying on my willingness to please, as well as my utter spinelessness, as its weaponry. By then, as a result of societal and familial influences, real or imagined, I viewed the phrase "I'm a people person" as code for "I have no definable skills." "I want to be an actress" equated to "I'm self-absorbed and delusional." Basically, anything short of conventional, left-brained pursuits had become, in my mind, the equivalent of running off to join the circus. And since I was born with an enlarged desire to garner approval from society, as well as from my law school–educated family, I certainly did not want to be perceived as the sword-swallowing bearded lady.

"You'd make a fine judge or professor or CEO one day," Dad and his parents often said to me, intending to convey a sincere compliment.

Aren't families *supposed* to encourage young girls to shatter glass ceilings in male-dominated professions? To kick ass and take names in courtrooms and boardrooms across America? Of course! I'm not complaining about my family's high aspirations for me—it's just that, in retrospect, I know I should have responded: "Thanks, but I don't really care about civil procedure. I just want to be on *Saturday Night Live*." And yet through absence of clarity or courage, or maybe both, I didn't say any such thing.

And anyway, as much as I'd absolutely loved being among the artsy types in the theater department, I knew I wasn't one of them. At theater parties, everywhere I looked, someone was experimenting with drugs or sexuality (or both), or doing a manic stand-up routine to an audience of three. And me? I was the Girl with Her Head on Straight. The Girl with a Boyfriend Back Home. I didn't have any interest in luxuriating in angst or drugs, or in "finding myself." I was the only person I knew who'd never even smoked pot, for Pete's sake.

I wasn't a thespian like my roommate Holly, who was angst-ridden and deep in a way I couldn't fathom; I was just sort of . . . faking it. But one day soon, if I continued down this gotta-be-me path, I worried, the jig would be up and I'd wind up with no marketable skills, serving "Adam and Eve on a Raft" at a truck stop forever.

At the time, I am sure, I couldn't have articulated any of this. But in retrospect, it's clear that my head had finally beaten the pulp out of my heart, after years of epic struggle. And so, for all of these reasons, I jumped the first train to Plan B and joined Brad in law school.

Goodbye, Judy.

Score one for the head.

Chapter 11

Although Brad and I had spent many a weekend together up to this point, living together full-time was an adjustment. I would go to the grocery store to buy what I thought was a week's worth of groceries, only to find that Brad had emptied the refrigerator a mere two days later. And since I'd never had a brother, I wasn't hip to all the pointless and imbecilic teasing that's second nature to boys.

Once, when there were two cookies left on a plate, I asked Brad for one of them.

"Sure," he said, and then he picked up both cookies, licked them with exaggerated gusto, and held them both out to me, a cocky grin on his handsome face. "Which one do you want?"

I was aghast. "You're an animal!"

He just laughed his silly, infectious laugh.

And Brad learned new things about me, too—like the fact that I was a somnambulatory lunatic.

"Honey, what are you doing?" he asked, dumbfounded, having awakened to find me gingerly patting a large houseplant in the corner of our bedroom.

"Shhhh!" I admonished with intensity. "You'll scare it!"

Brad turned on the bedroom light and said, "I'm pretty sure I'm not gonna scare a houseplant."

I awoke from my trance. "Oh," I said, bewildered. "I thought it was an injured German shepherd."

In addition to learning about my nighttime secrets, Brad discovered (as did I) that my Brooklyn-born mother's "from *da nay-buh-hood*" accent had tainted my speech since birth.

Sharon and I had visited our Brooklyn grandparents during many childhood summers, endlessly amusing ourselves with our simulations of that distinctive accent. My favorite pastime in the world was to sit in the muggy summer air on my grandparents' front porch ("the stoop") and, simply by sitting there, lure the neighborhood kids to me like moths to the flame. What Brooklynite could resist chatting with the visiting girl from California?

"Say *dwahg*," one of them would prompt, after a small crowd had formed.

"Dog," I'd answer politely, in my perfect Grace Kelly diction, my California-bred superiority wafting from every pore.

Hysterical laughter would ensue from the menagerie.

"Say *cwahffee*," one of the kids would shout.

"Coffee."

Peals of laughter.

"Say *mirr-uh*."

"Mirror."

Mass hysteria.

I amused *them?* Okay, I'd let them enjoy their alternate reality, even though I knew, without a doubt, that *they* were the
amusing ones.

And so, years later, when Brad and I finally shacked up and each
day brought a new revelation about the other person, I was blindsided
to learn that, despite my holier-than-thou tours of duty on that stoop
in Brooklyn, my movie-star pronunciation had been compromised at
the cellular level.

"Hand me the spatuler," I instructed Brad one morning as I
scrambled eggs for our breakfast.

"The *what?!*" he asked, an incredulous smile forming on his lips.

"The spatuler."

"It's called a spa-tu-la," Brad said, imbuing every syllable with
condescension.

"No, it isn't," I countered. *You idiot.*

"Yes, it is."

"No, it isn't." In a huff, I pulled out a big dictionary and slammed
it onto the kitchen counter. I was positive I was right. My mom was a
great cook, and I'd heard her use the word "spatuler" my whole life!

I flipped to the appropriate page of the dictionary and scanned
down the left column until . . . *I'll be damned, it's a spatula.*

There was no denying it: I was half Brooklyn-ese.

I had signed up with a temp agency and was assigned random office jobs—typing, answering phones, data entry—usually for a day at a time. After a few weeks, I got a plum assignment: organizing file cabinets for *a full week!* The best part was, if the employers liked me, they might extend my contract for three months. I'd be in the money.

The night before starting my new assignment, I went to bed plenty early to ensure optimum file-cabinet-organization readiness the following morning. About an hour after I'd drifted off to sleep, I dreamed I was standing on a train track with a train hurtling toward me at an alarming speed. The train light was rapidly advancing, but—oh no!—I was rooted to the middle of the track! To save myself, I leaped with abandon out of the way and into an adjacent thorny bush.

As it turned out, I actually made that life-or-death leap in the real world, too—off my bed and into my nearby closet. And right onto my face. Without breaking my fall, even a little bit. My face smashed right into the high-heeled shoes sitting at the bottom of my closet.

The next morning, as I arrived at my new temp job, I had a swollen shiner, scratches all over my face, and a broken blood vessel in my eye. *Hello, my name is Laura! Nice to meetcha!* How's that for a first impression? My new coworkers immediately asked me what on earth had happened to me. My response? The classic response of anyone feeling too embarrassed to admit a shameful truth: "I fell."

Now, I ask you, which do you think is a better sell to a new employer: "I have night terrors that cause me to leap out of bed and slam my face on a pile of shoes in the middle of the night" or

"I am the victim of brutal domestic abuse"? Apparently, I thought the latter. But letting an employer believe I had battered-woman syndrome turned out to be the wrong choice: Despite my expert filing work, the company did not renew my temp contract at the end of the week.

A couple months of sporadic temp work later, I finally landed a permanent job selling tours to Turkey, though I'd never been there. Brad got a job working for a famous yacht skipper who was preparing to compete in the America's Cup (a fancy-shmancy sailboat race, so we were told), even though Brad had never stepped foot aboard a yacht. Between my job selling Turkey tours and Brad's job promoting a highfalutin yacht race, he and I endured our year off before law school as the Couple with the Most Random Jobs on the Face of the Earth.

A few months after my high-heeled face-plant and shortly before the start of law school, my sixth sense was buzzing.

"Brad," I said, "if you're thinking of proposing to me, please don't. I love you so much, but I don't want to get married until I'm thirty. I don't want to break your heart."

When I came home from a rough day of selling tours to Turkey a couple weeks later, Brad had cleaned the little house. *Strange.* Next, I saw that he had prepared a steak dinner for us. *Impossible.* When, after dinner, Brad told me to close my eyes, I thought eagerly, *Dessert?* To my shock, though, he got down on one knee, ring in hand, and asked me to marry him.

Despite my clear directive of only a few weeks earlier, I did not hesitate in my answer: "Yes!"

Despite my tendency toward excitability and my nighttime visions of oncoming trains, Brad loved me.

Much later, when I had gathered my wits about me, I stipulated that I would take Brad's name on one condition: "You have to promise to always use the accent on the *é* in Roppé." I had noticed that Brad and other members of his family were lazy about their accenting—sometimes they accented, and sometimes they didn't. "With the accent on the *é*," I continued, "the name is exotic, sort of French sounding. Ro-*pay*. But without it, well, it's just 'Rope.'"

Brad agreed.

A year later, at the blowout bash following our fairytale wedding (a generous gift from Dad), our elegantly clad friends, most of whom had just finished their first grueling year of law school, devolved into sweaty heathens and partied like it was 1999.

As Brad and I departed the wedding reception, I drunkenly invited every single wedding guest I walked past to join us upstairs in our honeymoon suite, while Brad, walking two feet behind me, soberly *un*invited every single guest. When Brad and I arrived, as husband and wife, at the honeymoon suite overlooking the San Diego skyline, I looked around, confused.

"Where *is* everyone?"

Brad just laughed his silly laugh.

Chapter 12

After all of our oncologist shopping, Brad and I finally settled on Dr. Andrew Hampshire, an unassuming family man of my exact age, whose easy laugh struck me as an anomaly for someone in his line of work.

Dr. Hampshire was warm and instantly likable, even when he was the bearer of bad news. And, most impressive to Brad and me, he was a dead ringer—both physically and temperamentally—for the best-friend character, Wilson, on the medical drama *House* (who, strangely enough, also happens to be an oncologist). Brad and I loved that show, so it was a no-brainer.

In addition to reminding us of one of our favorite TV doctors, Dr. Hampshire was ridiculously knowledgeable about cancer, and particularly about this newly discovered villain on the scene, triple negative breast cancer. He'd read all the latest studies and been to the latest triple-negative summits (facts we discovered when Brad, who'd initially been wary of Dr. Hampshire's youth, interrogated him in a manner befitting an episode of *Law & Order*).

And, best of all, Dr. Hampshire, who much later insisted we call him Andy, understood our complicated sense of humor (i.e., that it was Brad's job to make jokes and mine to laugh at them). Indeed, despite the serious context of most of our discussions with Dr. Hampshire, visits with him inevitably devolved into chortles of laughter on all sides.

But at my first appointment, as Brad and I searched for a doctor who could turn our world right side up again, we had not yet eased into the comfort of our cancer-comedy routine. No, at our first oncology appointment, Dr. Hampshire was warm but all business, matter-of-factly detailing the chemotherapy I would endure over the course of the next several months.

"We have to hit the cancer with the strongest chemo drugs available because it's so aggressive," he explained.

"Bring it on," I told him, full of false bravado. And, handing him a picture of the girls, I added, "Here's why I need to get better. I'll do whatever it takes."

Dr. Hampshire looked at the photo—I mean, he *really* looked at it—and nodded. He had a wife and three young kids of his own. His daughter's poem about a nature hike with her heroic dad was hanging on the wall behind his head, I noticed.

"If you were my wife," Dr. Hampshire said, and he looked right into my eyes, "I'd recommend this exact chemo regimen. It's best to do everything in your power against this thing now, so you never second-guess yourself later."

My life was in this man's hands. And he would care for me as if I were his own beloved wife.

Dr. Hampshire shifted his gaze to Brad, who nodded.

Brad trusted him. An understanding had passed between them. We'd found our man.

Brad handed Dr. Hampshire a copy of my album. "And there's also this." His voice quavered, just a little bit. "She wrote all the songs." Brad looked over at me, his face awash in tenderness and pride.

Dr. Hampshire scrutinized the CD cover, looking surprised. "So, you're a rock star?" he asked me, grinning.

"Well, no, not really." I'm pretty sure I batted my eyelashes shamelessly at him. "But when this is all over, I'm going over to England to film a music video!" I sounded a little bit maniacal, even to myself.

Dr. Hampshire was gracious. "Laura," he said, a fountain of reassurance, "you're going to film that music video. You're going to be just fine."

I clenched my jaw. *Damn straight.*

Thank you, Dr. Hampshire.

Chapter 13

Newlyweds Brad and Laura Roppé sat side by side on the first day of Constitutional Law class. The professor looked down at his class list, taking roll in alphabetical order:

"Bradley . . . *Rope?*"

"Ro-*pay*," Brad corrected. "Here."

The professor smiled at Brad and then looked down at his list, searching for the next name. "Laura . . . *Rope?*"

"Ro-*pay*. Here."

The entire classroom erupted in laughter.

At the end of my first year in law school, I was number one in our class. Brad, a big grin on his face, told anyone who'd listen, "I'm sick of her riding my coattails all the time."

Two years later, as Brad and I graduated from law school together, hand in hand, I'd slipped to number two.

"Number two? Loser!" Brad needled me, laughing. "I knew you were riding my coattails all along."

In any event, being a "loser" didn't seem to hurt my employment prospects: I had my pick of jobs at graduation time. Without a thought, off I went to work as a civil litigator at my top pick, one of the most prestigious law firms in San Diego. Hypnotized by the world of high salaries and pretty offices, I didn't stop to think, even once, *What do I want?* I just plucked a low-hanging plum off the tree and took a big, juicy bite, without considering whether I even liked plums at all.

It didn't take long before I figured out that *studying to become* a lawyer was a helluva lot more fun than *being* a lawyer. My daily life became about people fighting over money—whether relating to a real estate deal gone bad, a business contract turned sideways, or a busted employment relationship. Every day was all about money, money, money and fighting, fighting, fighting. My daily life was other people's problems—OPP—and no, I wasn't "down with OPP."

The swanky law firm where I worked was right out of the movie *The Firm*—sleek marble tables, plush leather chairs, and floor-to-ceiling views of the skyline. Elegant older men with silver hair and designer suits cut through the quiet hallways, their assistants twittering and trailing behind.

I worked long days, well into every evening, and most weekends, too. I never said no when someone asked me to do any task, no matter how big or small. I kept track of time worked on my cases in six-minute increments, to be billed to the client—the system known in the law field as keeping track of "billable hours." At the end of the first year, I felt immense satisfaction at being the attorney who'd logged the most billable hours in my entire firm. I was a workhorse.

Consistent with my impeccable, precise surroundings, my suits were tailored to perfection, hugging the stick-thin frame I had worked so hard to achieve with a daily five-mile run and strict no-fat diet. Everything about me screamed "type A," right down to my A-line bob.

The three "elders" of the firm could not have been more different: Doug, the managing partner, had a singsongy way of asking, "How're you?" as he passed in the hall; Gary, the top rainmaker, was formal and exacting and intimidating as hell; and Curt, the swashbuckler, was pure, unadulterated masculinity—I was pretty sure I ovulated every time he entered the room.

The women partners were especially interesting to me as I tried to imagine my future as a partner at this firm. June was an old broad in the tradition of Bette Davis, calling 'em like she saw 'em, smokin' and drinkin' whiskey after work with the big boys. Sue was a billable-hours machine, churning out briefs and depositions at such a rapid-fire pace, I didn't have more than a five-minute conversation with her over the course of eight years. Her manic work ethic did not appeal to me, though I was following right in her footsteps.

The woman who influenced me most was my mentor, Janice, who was like no one else I'd ever met in my life—a tornado. She was an African American woman who, through sheer tenacity, had risen to the esteemed rank of partner at a major law firm in her early forties. But she hadn't accomplished that feat by staying on a traditional path;

no, she had gone the opposite direction: When every other attorney was dressed in conservative gray, Janice wore electric pink St. John knits, flashy scarves, and Prada heels. She was all woman, daring everyone in the room not to notice her. She was charming, flat-out stunning, and funny. She cracked jokes, even in the courtroom. And, man, could she bring in new clients. She was fascinating to me.

One day, Janice buzzed me and told me to come into her office. When I walked in, there was Eric Allen, one of the NFL's premier defensive backs. Janice knew I was a huge football fan and that I was enamored of Eric Allen's athletic prowess (okay, his gorgeous eyes).

As I approached this Adonis-like man to shake his hand, a high-pitched squeal caught in my throat, and I worried it would escape from my mouth. *That wouldn't be very lawyerlike, Laura. Keep it together.*

"Laura, this is Eric Allen." Janice motioned to me. "Eric, this is my associate Laura."

Eric Allen extended his hand, and I shook it. *Way too hard.*

And then, in a staccato voice that was three octaves lower than my normal speaking voice, I barked out, "Nice to meet you!" *Ugh.* I had overcompensated for the squeal I had tried to suppress. It was my trying-to-seem-professional voice, only on major steroids. I sounded like the drill sergeant in *Full Metal Jacket*.

"Nice to meet you, too," Mr. Allen replied generously. But his amused smile was undeniable.

Janice heckled me about the Eric Allen Incident for years after that. And, I had to admit, it was pretty damned funny. My embarrassment was well worth it, though: Even when Janice was laughing at me, which was often, I gloried in the warm light of her attention.

She and I sat in her office many a night after everyone else had gone home for the day, talking endlessly about "our dreams," though I can't for the life of me remember what I contributed to those conversations. Janice told me about how she wanted to own a law firm one day and create a place where lawyers could find balance in their lives. And what were my dreams? Well, I just adopted hers. "Me, too" was my mantra—the easiest and only thing to say, since I'd stopped dreaming for myself.

Janice and I were working on a case as cocounsel with a huge national law firm in Washington, D.C. This particular litigation involved writing endless legal briefs, the sheer volume of which was too much for any one person to accomplish. The writing tasks were therefore divided up between me and the associate at the other law firm, a guy named Alan. Alan and I spoke on the phone almost every day to integrate our portions of the legal briefs. Based on his voice, which was sort of nebbishy and passive, I had a visual image of him that popped into my head every time we spoke: a tall, skinny white guy with brown hair and glasses. A stereotypical accountant. Or, I guess, more aptly, a corporate lawyer.

One day while Alan and I were on one of our many phone calls to talk about our never-ending writing tasks, he told me a story about a lawyer in his firm who always interjected into any conversation the fact that he'd been on the law review at his Ivy League law school. In a mockingly pompous voice, Alan imitated the man to demonstrate his point: "'That reminds me of when I was on law review . . . '"

We both chuckled. "Oh, how annoying," I said. "I hate it when people never stop bragging about their resumes. Especially when their accomplishments aren't recent."

"You're right," Alan agreed. "A person can't rest on past accomplishments forever. You have to keep growing, getting better."

"Totally!"

And then Alan's tone shifted. He sounded contemplative. "Honestly, I worry sometimes I dwell too much on my NFL days . . . "

His NFL days? I didn't hear anything Alan said beyond that phrase. What the hell? Alan had played in the NFL? My mind was reeling. *Was he a kicker? Does. Not. Compute.*

"Alan, go back a minute. What do you mean, your 'NFL days'?"

"Oh, yeah," he said nonchalantly. "I played in the NFL."

Silence hung in the air for a beat while that sank in. "What position?"

"Defensive back. For the Eagles."

What?! I was stupefied. I had been talking to this guy every day for months! Throughout that time, my mental image of him had become so fixed in my mind, I was finding it hard to readjust. *He must not be so skinny,* I thought.

About a month later, Alan and the other lawyers from his firm paid a visit to my firm's San Diego office.

Janice buzzed me. "Come to the conference room," she said. "Alan wants to meet you."

After months of talking on the phone and working so hard on our legal briefs together, it would be a pleasure to finally meet Alan face-to-face.

When I entered the conference room, Janice was standing next to a man who could not possibly have been Alan. But then she said, "Laura, this is Alan."

I smiled. Alan wasn't tall and skinny. And he didn't wear glasses or look like an accountant, either. In fact, he was handsome, and muscled, and masculine. Oh, and one other thing: *Alan was black.* I burst out laughing as I hugged my long-distance friend. And after a few moments of warm conversation, I felt comfortable enough to admit to him, "You know, Alan, this whole time, I thought you were a tall, skinny white guy with glasses!"

Alan laughed heartily. "That's okay, Laura," he said. "I thought you were a short, fat Latina."

Even through my laughter, I immediately recognized the important lesson: *Books don't always match their covers.*

When the time came for me to defend a corporate client in my first big trial, I was thrilled when I caught our adversary, the company's former employee, in an outright lie on the witness stand. I was Matlock! Victory would be mine!

But when the jury read their verdict a week later, they had found in favor of the former employee and against my big client. Not only that, but they had further found that my client had "acted with malice" in firing this gentleman, meaning the jury could now consider an award of punitive damages, the granddaddy of damages awards—a potential catastrophe for my client.

The judge scheduled the punitive-damages phase of the trial for the following day.

That night, I couldn't sleep a wink. I was flabbergasted that I'd lost. I had believed in my case, but the jury hadn't believed in me. And now the jury was poised to render a verdict, in perhaps the millions of dollars, to punish my client. I thought I was going to be sick.

The next day, I had dark circles under my eyes and my face was tight.

I stepped in front of the jury—the same jury who had just condemned my client the day before—and pleaded my case for them to deny punitive damages. As I spoke, I could feel my knobby knees knocking together underneath my gray pencil skirt.

When the jury returned its verdict later that afternoon—glory be!— they awarded a pittance, hardly anything at all. I thought I might pass out from relief. I made my way into the hallway outside the courtroom, where I was allowed to speak with the jury now that the trial was over.

"Laura," the foreperson said to me (and I recall distinctly that she addressed me by my first name), "we hated your client." Everyone added their vocal agreement to that sentiment. "But we loved you."

Another juror added, "You're so funny!"

More vocal agreement, and warm smiles.

The foreperson continued, "You looked so nervous this morning, we decided we didn't want to ruin your career by awarding big punitive damages against your client."

Excuse me? I was grateful for their mercy, of course. The verdict had been a huge relief. But this wasn't my idea of justice—this was a crapshoot!

In an instant, I realized something that shook me to my core: I was living my life, both personally and professionally, in pursuit of external approval. And that dangling carrot, I suddenly understood, was a prize as fickle as the wind.

The whole affair left me wondering what the hell I was doing with my life.

As the years passed, I continued working the crazy hours required of a litigation associate. I worked and worked and worked, and received bonuses and assurances that I was "on partnership track." And though I relished the praise, as well as my time with Janice and other friends I'd made at the firm, I became overwhelmed with the stress of my job.

Every morning as I drove in to work, my stomach turned to knots. As I sat down at my desk to start each day, I gave myself a pep talk about facing the confrontations that awaited me. *This is what they pay you to do,* I'd tell myself before picking up the phone to call a particularly rude opposing attorney.

Night terrors regularly interrupted my sleep (and Brad's). One night, I turned to Brad in the middle of the night, waking him from a dead sleep, and shouted at him, my heart racing and my eyes bulging, "Who *are* you?!" In the morning, my throat was raw.

Year-end bonuses and incentives didn't motivate me anymore. A bone tiredness overtook me.

"I feel like I have a terminal illness," I lamented to Brad one day during a grueling case.

Supernatural prophesy yet again? Nah. I was twenty-eight years old, and as far as I was concerned, I was immortal. But I felt like my soul had been sucked dry of all moisture, like a sponge that's turned rock-hard sitting too long on a sink ledge. No, I didn't think I was actually terminally ill; what I meant to say was, I was *terminally tired*.

"Hang in there, Buddy," Brad consoled me. "You'll be fine."

Chapter 14

Countdown to chemo: two weeks.

By this time, I had long since passed the denial phase. Now, I was just petrified. It was now a reality that, yes, bad things could happen to me. A doctor had already called with unthinkable news. He had said "cancer," and he had been talking about me. And then he had added words like "rare" and "aggressive" and "triple negative." I had thought something was impossible, but it had proved entirely possible—and not in a *Charlie and the Chocolate Factory* sort of way.

At my next oncology appointment, Dr. Hampshire told me, in no uncertain terms, that I would lose all my hair during chemo. Everywhere. Without a doubt.

"Well, you never know," I countered. "Maybe I will and maybe I won't." I ran my fingers through my long, thick hair.

"No, you will," Dr. Hampshire said matter-of-factly. "With this particular chemo drug [a beast called Adriamycin], there is no doubt you'll lose your hair. One hundred percent of the people lose one hundred percent of their hair, one hundred percent of the time." He didn't want me to hold out false hopes.

I'd come to expect, and appreciate, Dr. Hampshire's unflinching honesty. It was best to know what I was up against. I looked at Brad and sighed. I liked having hair. A whole lot.

"Don't worry, honey. It'll grow back," Brad said with a sympathetic smile, and he kissed me on the forehead.

Cancer might take my hair, I thought, *but that's all it's getting.*

A week later, my sister, Sharon, accompanied me to my neighborhood hair salon. I had decided I would lose my hair on my own terms and donate it to Locks of Love, a wigmaker for children with cancer. And selfishly, I also figured it would be somehow less traumatizing to lose short hair.

"If I feel like we're making a documentary, I can get through it," I told Sharon. "Never stop taking pictures." Thus, as the hairdresser cut my hair to pixie length, Sharon imitated a photojournalist, snapping endless photos of me. I made silly faces and gave her two thumbs up (my patented "stay positive" pose), and we laughed and laughed.

Sharon has always been my touchstone, through every form of heartbreak and catastrophe. As little girls, when our black cat, Kitty, went missing for over a week, Sharon and I cleaved to each other, stoking each other's waning faith that Kitty was all right. After a tip from our neighbor that Kitty might have met his maker in the street, Sharon and I crept outside, trembling and holding on to each other for dear life.

Sure enough, we discovered what used to be our Kitty, now

reduced to a furry lump on the asphalt. My brain could not accept that the mound before my eyes was my beloved Kitty, but Sharon understood. She broke into a horrified wail, clutching my slender body with the full force of her grief.

Sharon's hysteria jarred me from my stupor—just as our kind neighbor swept Kitty into a dustpan—and I started screaming, too, almost collapsing into Sharon's arms in my horror.

To this day, our shared grief at having found Kitty-Lump in the street is one of the defining vignettes of our sisterhood: Sharon and I were there to prop each other up through thick and thin, no matter what.

And now, just as I had done throughout my entire life, I was holding on to Sharon yet again, though perhaps not physically in this instance, as the hairdresser relieved my head of all its hair in anticipation of my imminent chemotherapy.

When I approached the front counter to pay for the haircut, still laughing with Sharon and making my "stay positive" thumbs up, the salon manager wouldn't take my money.

"It's a gift," she said. "We just wish you a speedy recovery."

In that moment, the full weight of my predicament fell on my head like a wayward theater sandbag from an episode of *Scooby-Doo* ("and I would have succeeded, too, if it wasn't for you meddling kids!"). Strange as it may sound, I had actually forgotten what had led me to the hair salon in the first place. I had tricked myself into thinking I was just a normal girl getting a "whole new me" haircut—as part of a midlife crisis, perhaps? Or maybe on a dare? But the salon manager's kind gift reminded me: *No, I'm a cancer patient.*

I started to cry. Sharon did, too. We collapsed into each other's arms, just as we did when we discovered that poor Kitty had gone off to take an eternal nap.

It was the first stamp in my cancer passport.

When I went to pick up the girls from school later that day, I wore a straw hat so they couldn't see my new, short hair. I wanted them to be able to react to it privately, away from their friends.

I waited outside Chloe's first-grade classroom, reminding myself to take deep breaths.

"Hi, Mom," Chloe said when she emerged, her Dora the Explorer backpack slung over her shoulder. "Hey, your hair's gone." And then she started rambling on about her day.

Well, that went well.

But when Sophie made her way out of her third-grade classroom, her face turned pale the moment she saw me. Tears filled her eyes, and she tilted her head back to keep them from spilling down her cheeks.

"Baby," I assured her, "it's okay."

"Don't talk to me," Sophie hissed between clenched teeth, and she marched ahead as if she didn't know me.

As I followed Sophie's angry little body to the car, my lips were trembling.

During the short drive to our house in our minivan, I could not find words. Every time I started to speak, my throat closed up and nothing came out. We drove in silence (and by "silence," I mean that Sophie and I did not speak; Chloe, on the other hand, chatted non-stop about her day at school—about her boyfriend, Jackson; about her latest *Geronimo Stilton* book; about how her teacher had broken her toe on her coffee table—all the while not disturbed one iota that not a wisp of hair was peeking out from under Mommy's hat).

When we got home, Sophie burst into tears. "Why did you *do* that?" she demanded.

"Baby," I said, "I'm so sorry. The doctor says I'm going to lose my hair, and I wanted to beat it to the punch." I started to cry, too.

Sophie was pissed. This was so embarrassing, so mean, so awful. How *could* I? Why was I *doing* this to her?

"I'm sorry," I sighed. I sat down on the couch and took off my hat.

Sophie's eyes widened. "Oh my God," she gasped.

"What is it?" I was worried. I touched my head.

Sophie sat down next to me. "Mom, that's actually pretty cute."

Oh, geez, she scared me. "Really?"

"Yeah. Really."

I hugged her. "Thank you, Soph-a-loph."

Chapter 15

Brad had always been moony-eyed about having kids; if I'd said yes, we would have started trying for a baby on our honeymoon. But I'd never given him the green light. I had invested a lot of time and money in law school, and once I began working, having a baby would have cramped my billable-hours style.

Even more than worrying about my career, I wasn't sure I wanted children at all. As a teen, I'd done my share of baby-sitting to earn extra cash, but, although the kids in my care were cutie pies, I had never thought, *Oh, I can't wait to have kids of my own one day.* Throughout my twenties, I'd never clamored to hold other people's babies (though I did hold them, so as not to arouse suspicion about my lack of maternal instincts). My "oohs" and "ahhs" at baby showers about itty-bitty baby clothes had been forced, a total sham. I was missing the baby gene. I could easily envision a fulfilling life filled with Brad, work, and my crazy-ass dog.

Then one evening, at age twenty-eight, I popped into the grocery store to pick up dinner after a long day at work. As I waited in line at the checkout stand, shifting my weight from one foot to the other in my stiletto heels, my tired eyes settled on a baby boy sitting in the grocery cart ahead of me. He wasn't wearing any shoes, and his fat toes looked impossibly tiny. I hadn't examined baby toes before. They were darling! *Awww,* I thought, for possibly the first time in my life. When I looked up from those little sausage toes, the baby had fixed his gaze on me. His eyes were crystal blue. *Awww,* I thought yet again. And then he smiled—a big, innocent, goofy smile that sent a thunderbolt zinging through my heart. *Gimme that baby.*

At home, I marched through the front door and beelined to the bathroom, calling for Brad to meet me there. When he arrived, a question on his face, I raised my packet of birth control pills into the air, like an Olympic diver about to swan-dive off the high platform. Brad raised his eyebrows at me, not understanding, and just as he opened his mouth to ask what was going on, I plopped the packet of pills into the metal trash can with a *clank.* There was a brief silence as Brad processed what he was witnessing. An instant later, pure joy washed over his face.

For months after my triumphant offering to the fertility gods, poor Brad would pick up the phone at work, only to be greeted by my screeching voice on the other end: "I'm *ovulating!* Meet me at home *right now!"* Two weeks later, I'd sit down on the toilet and pee on a stick, holding my breath and willing a pink line to show up. But it never came.

I continued to rack up the billable hours at work. Every day blended into the next, except that I had begun to wear a different brightly colored scarf around my neck each day—just like Janice did—though the look was ridiculous on me. (If my fourteen-year-old self had gotten a glimpse of her twenty-eight-year-old self in a fuchsia suit with gold buttons and a flowered scarf tied in a slipknot around her neck, she would have thrown her head back and bawled, "For the love of God, no!")

I would stand in my office on the twenty-first floor, leaning my forehead against the floor-to-ceiling window, and gaze down at the ant-people below as they hustled and bustled across the crowded streets. *Every one of them exists because a woman got pregnant,* I would think.

Mom had gotten pregnant with my sister the first time she'd ever had sex (with my dad, at age eighteen), and she'd pounded this fact into my head and Sharon's repeatedly, urgently, throughout our teen-age years. As a result, my entire life I'd believed, without a shadow of a doubt, that one (itty-bitty) act of unprotected sex would result in pregnancy every single time. It was an absolute, proven fact.

So why wasn't I Fertile Myrtle, like Mom?

I'd heard plenty of stories of vacation-induced pregnancies, so off Brad and I went on a ski vacation with friends. After a day of skiing, I made my way to the hotel's fancy spa, where I drank cucumber water and flipped through *Spa* magazine while awaiting my massage appointment.

"Laura . . . *Rope?*"

"Yes. Ro-*pay*. Hi."

My masseuse, a broad-shouldered German named Helga (actually, I can't remember her real name, but she will always be Helga to me), led me to a dimly lit room, where I purred like a cat as I crawled onto the massage table. Helga drizzled oil on my back and began kneading my tight muscles. After a few minutes, she graduated to grinding her elbows into my back.

"Your tension is the worst I have ever seen," she chastised me in a harsh German accent.

Was she serious? The *worst* she'd ever seen? *C'mon.*

"So much stress!" she accused again.

Was she expecting me to say something here?

After a few more minutes, Helga grunted, "You are trying to have a baby, yes?"

What? That got my attention. "Yes." *How did she know?*

And then Helga dropped the bomb: "How do you expect to take care of a baby *when you cannot take care of yourself?*" She emitted a loud hissing noise that ended with "Tsk-tsk."

I was floored.

I paid for the massage (which, in this case, felt like a punch in the gut) and shuffled back to my hotel room. *I do take care of myself!* Helga's words had cut like a knife. *Am I unworthy of having a child?*

Back at the room, I told Brad about what Helga had said, and he told me not to worry about it. "During my massage, she told me I was a merman in a past life," he laughed.

But I *did* worry about it. Could there be a connection between my inability to get pregnant and the stress I was experiencing on the job? Was my body really the most stressed out Helga had *ever* seen? Her words continued to sting.

At home a few days later, I opened the phone book and scheduled a month's worth of weekly appointments with the nearest massage therapist. *I'll show you, Helga.*

Two months later, having dutifully attended regular massage sessions over the past several weeks, I sat down on the toilet yet again with a pregnancy test—wishing, hoping, and praying for a pink line to appear. And then . . . *oh* . . . *my* . . . *God.* There it was.

I ran out of the bathroom and pounced on Brad, who'd been fast asleep in bed, almost giving him a heart attack—which would have been a calamitous turn of events under the circumstances.

"Wake up, Buddy! Wake up!" I shouted, tears springing into my eyes. "We did it! We're gonna have a baby!"

What I didn't realize then was that I'd totally and completely missed Helga's point. I'd been so myopically focused on achieving that little pink line, I'd missed the Big Picture. Helga hadn't intended to enlighten me about how to board the *Baby Express;* she had wanted me to learn to appreciate the glorious views from the slow bus on the scenic route. If only I'd been able to understand what Helga was actually saying—that respect for the mind-body connection was the key to a healthy *life,* and not just a means of achieving my pregnancy goal—perhaps things might have turned out differently for me. Perhaps if I'd been capable of hearing the rallying cry of my knotted-up body, if I'd been humble enough to comprehend that my beleaguered pretzel body was shouting urgently at me, I might have avoided its exasperated, and inevitably violent, revolt nine years later.

But really, even if I'd known way back then that my body would eventually overthrow the existing regime in a bloody palace coup, I would have thrown my head back and laughed, "Let them eat cake!"— because at that moment, I was in mommy-to-be heaven. I was going to have a baby! And nothing else—*absolutely nothing else in the whole world*—mattered one little bit.

For the next five months, my violent daily heaving made me giddy, confirming that I was really, truly, not-imagining-this pregnant. Brad and I posted a track-each-day-of-your-pregnancy calendar on the refrigerator door so we could follow the minutia of the baby's development. *The baby is the size of a bean! The baby has arm buds! The baby is the size of a plum!* Brad, a man who never did any grocery shopping or cooking, ever, came home one evening with a raw ginger root to make a nausea-abating tea he'd read about online. At night, he massaged my aching back and feet. On weekends, we shopped for cribs and diaper-changing tables.

In the twentieth week of my pregnancy, we learned from a sonogram that our little bean was, in fact, a baby girl. *A daddy's girl! A Baby Sophie.*

I often dreamed about giving birth to our Sophie: Immediately following her birth, the doctor would place Sophie in my arms and I would kiss her little face, crying tears of joy. One night, the birth dream started as usual. But when I looked down to kiss the baby's little face, I was surprised to find I was not holding a baby; instead, I was holding a German shepherd puppy. I was crestfallen.

"Oh," I said in my dream, disappointed. "I was hoping for a *human* baby."

"Well, just keep trying," the doctor reassured me. "You just might get a human baby next time."

Relieved, and, frankly, still pretty happy—I mean, the puppy was adorable—I proceeded to kiss and cuddle my new puppy. Better luck next time!

When I woke up, I tried to understand the meaning of this strange dream. Did it mean I was ready to love my baby unconditionally? Or maybe I was projecting my love for Crazy Buster onto my unborn child. Or maybe, just maybe, my subconscious was telling me that I was not yet ready to graduate from dogs to babies.

I hoped to God it wasn't Door No. 3.

Sharon was pregnant, too, though it was her second time at the rodeo.

"I'm so big!" I exclaimed as she and I lay in bed together, comparing our watermelon-size bellies.

"I'm bigger," Sharon declared, and it wasn't clear if she was boasting or bemoaning.

And she was right. You see, Sharon was a shoo-in to win the whose-belly-is-bigger contest, because, although her due date was two months later than mine, her belly was filled with three times the number of babies.

Yes, Sharon was pregnant with triplets.

Yet the day after my due date had come and gone, I sat at Sharon's hospital bedside—she'd been admitted for regular infusions designed to delay premature labor—and had the nerve to complain, "This baby's never gonna come!"

Sharon—who had been hooked up to hospital machines and separated from her husband and two-year-old daughter—had the grace to laugh and roll her eyes along with me.

"Hang in there," she said. She looked so tired, but she smiled at me warmly.

When I arrived home from visiting Sharon in the hospital, I called her immediately, ready to heap another stack of complaints on my already rising pile.

But, to my surprise, a nurse answered Sharon's phone.

"Sharon's been rushed to the delivery room. She just delivered her babies."

I gasped. Sharon's due date was over two months away!

Oh, labor must have come on in a flash! I had been there just forty minutes before. A chill went down my spine.

I waddled frantically back to my car and raced back to the hospital. As I ran through the hospital front doors, breathless and clutching my belly (which had started contracting erratically because of the stress), a crowd of hospital staffers descended upon me, ushering me into a wheelchair.

"Who's your doctor?" they wanted to know. "Do you want us to call your husband?"

"No! No!" I shouted, waving away their helping hands. "I'm not in labor! I need to see my sister!"

I was on the verge of panic.

By the time I got to the delivery room, my sister's triplets—two boys and a girl—were already nestled in Plexiglas incubators, hooked up to monitors and wires. Born eleven weeks premature and weighing almost three pounds each, the newborns looked like animatronic Yoda-babies. Thankfully, the doctors said they'd all be fine.

Sharon looked pale but beatific.

Mom had already arrived and was talking nonstop, her standard reaction in times of stress.

My sister is a mother of four, I marveled, gazing at the babies' sixty combined fingers and toes, Mom's yakkity-yakking fading into white noise in the background.

Sixteen hours later, our Sophie made her grand entrance, looking as if she could squash all three of her preemie cousins with one chubby fist, or, alternatively, gobble them up as a midmorning snack.

Chapter 16

Now that my diagnosis and treatment plan had been confirmed by an actual oncologist, as opposed to "Dr. Brad," I decided to do some research online to find out what I was up against. I clicked on an article describing chemotherapy in detail: It is not a "targeted" cancer treatment, the article said. Chemo drugs seek out and destroy fast-growing cells of any type, including cancer cells—but also cells of the bone marrow, oral mucus membrane, linings of the stomach and intestine, and hair follicles. Due to the shotgun nature of chemo, the website explained, a chemo patient may experience lots of side effects, including fatigue, nausea, vomiting, loss of appetite, mouth sores, hair loss, premature menopause, bone loss, low red-blood-cell counts, low white-blood-cell counts, diarrhea, and constipation. And leukemia.

What? I could get leukemia from chemotherapy?

I threw my hands up into the air. And then I put my head on the desk. It was all so doomsday, I just didn't want to know. I didn't want any more information, I decided; what I wanted was support.

I navigated to the only triple-negative website I could find—for an organization called the Triple Negative Breast Cancer Foundation—and was momentarily paralyzed by the shocking array of pink ribbons that littered the site.

I saw a heading for "message boards" and clicked on the link. Wow, there were a gazillion postings. *So many women dealing with this crap.* Women had posted messages to each other covering every aspect of the disease and its treatment—surgery, hair loss, metallic tastes caused by the chemo drugs, nerve damage in extremities, depression. It was overwhelming. My predicament seemed insurmountable.

After reading other ladies' posts for quite some time, alternately biting my lip and wiping away tears from my cheeks, I did something I'd never done before on any website in my life: I posted a message—not to anyone in particular, but more to the universe at large. Was there anybody out there? I felt an undeniable urge to connect with someone else going through exactly what I was experiencing.

"I was recently diagnosed with TNBC," I wrote, tears welling up in my eyes. "I will start chemo soon." I paused. What did I really want to say? "I'm scared," I continued. And it was the truth. "Is there anyone out there? I need a friend."

With a heavy sigh, I wiped the tears for one last time, turned off the computer, and flopped into the warm bed next to Brad, who was already fast asleep.

The next morning, I awoke to find a reply message in my inbox.

It was from Jane, a recently diagnosed, forty-year-old woman from Sheffield, England.

"I'm scared, too," Jane wrote. "I'll be your friend, if you'll be mine."

Eureka!

I immediately sent Jane an email telling her how excited I was to have found her. She happened to be online at that very moment, and replied right back. A lengthy, giddy email exchange between us ensued, during which we discovered that Jane and I were both scheduled to undergo our first chemotherapy infusions *on the exact same day,* a few weeks later. We agreed to be each other's TNBC buddies.

"I feel like I have had a bit of a weight lifted from my shoulders, just knowing you are there," Jane wrote. "I am really thrilled that you want to take this journey with me and I look forward to us 'holding hands' across the pond as we both take our first trepidatious steps into chemo and beyond."

"You have made a big difference for me, too," I replied. "Thank you for holding my hand. I am squeezing it right now."

Over the next few weeks, Jane and I prepared ourselves for chemo. Even though we were embarking on our respective battles on separate continents, it felt like we were arm in arm. In a flurry of emails, we compared the different chemo drugs our oncologists had recommended, traded practical tips we'd read about how to combat chemo side effects, and sent each other links to websites that donated head scarves and hats. We divulged personal-ad-type details about ourselves: "I love reading, listening to music, socialising, and being with my family—however much they drive me nuts," Jane wrote. In response to my descriptions of Brad and the girls, Jane wrote to me about her husband, Adam, and two-year-old daughter, Natasha.

We gave each other pep talks. Jane cheered me on: "You must not let this bloody disease ruin your dreams! It may feel like it is in control of you but you can be in control of it!"

And I replied, "I am one hundred percent here for you, squeezing your hand, sending you positive vibes. You can do this. The cancer won't know what hit it!"

We vented and complained about things we couldn't reveal to anyone else, lest we cause worry or offense. Jane wrote, "I had a bit of a wobble the other day. I couldn't stop crying and crying."

For my part, I bristled against "staying positive" all the time, the universally accepted mantra for defeating cancer: "I am told 10,000 times a day to 'stay positive.' Yes, of course. But I was not 'positive' 24/7 before cancer, and I'm not going to be positive 24/7 after cancer. I believe completely in a positive attitude, no doubt. But I was already a positive person. And I got cancer."

Jane agreed and suggested we get matching T-shirts bearing the slogan STAY POSITIVE, with two thumbs up. We just understood each other.

I lamented Brad's suffering: "How is your husband? I have seen mine cry more in the past week than in the twenty-three years I've known him. It's devastating. He keeps saying he wishes he could do it for me. . . . " To which Jane replied that, strangely enough, her husband hadn't cried at all. I chalked it up to Adam's (very) British stiff upper lip.

And then, in one of our email exchanges, I fortuitously addressed

Jane as "My Dearest Jane," and noted that this was how Miss Elizabeth Bennet in Jane Austen's classic *Pride and Prejudice* had always addressed her elder sister, Jane, in letters. Well, that certainly touched a chord with Jane: "Do you like *Pride and Prejudice*?!" she wrote, and I could hear her exuberance through cyberspace. "I love P&P! Did you get the BBC's version of it with Jennifer Ehle and Colin Firth over there? Being a bit of a romantic at heart, my most favourite part is when, although he gets rebuffed, Mr. Darcy says to Elizabeth: 'In vain I have struggled. It will not do. My feelings will not be repressed. You must allow me to tell you how ardently I admire and love you.' Oh, be still my beating heart!"

I'd found my soul mate! I didn't know anyone, other than Mom and Sharon, who'd even *seen* the BBC version of *Pride and Prejudice*, let alone adored it like I did.

Thanks to my mom, I'd been a period-drama junkie my whole life.

"Come on in," Mom had said to Sharon and me during those first uncertain months after her divorce from Dad, holding up the corner of her bedspread.

And Sharon and I had crammed into her warm bed, transfixed by Scarlett O'Hara and Rhett Butler in *Gone with the Wind*—a life-altering movie that inspired me to randomly shoehorn "fiddle dee dee" into countless conversations for the better part of a year.

Years later, when Sharon and I were in our twenties, the three of us had crammed into Mom's bed yet again, this time swooning over all six hours of the BBC's *Pride and Prejudice*, starring the scorching Colin Firth as Mr. Darcy. Since that first viewing, I had become addicted, regularly watching all six hours in one sitting. I knew it was unhealthy, but I just couldn't stop.

And now here was another woman afflicted with *both* triple negative breast cancer and *Pride and Prejudice* fever, just like me! What were the odds?

"My Dearest Jane," I replied, "yes, I am obsessed with *Pride and Prejudice.* I have seen the BBC version probably twenty full times and I am not exaggerating. People in the U.S. are not obsessed with this; most do not know it exists, so there is no accounting for it. My favorite part is also his first proposal. I would have said 'Yes!' I wouldn't care if he had insulted my family or said his feelings violated his judgment and social situation. I would have said 'yes' and then tackled him and had my way with him right then and there."

And thus, through a shared belief that Mr. Darcy's proposal to Miss Bennet was, without a doubt, the single most romantic moment in cinematic history, a friendship born from cancer transcended into an unbreakable sisterhood.

Chapter 17

Before I had my baby, I envisioned my life as a world map. My marriage was North America; my career was Europe; my family, Asia; and my friends, Australia. When I became pregnant, I assumed my future baby would fit right into my world map, like a thumbtack marking a city. My baby would be . . . Rome, perhaps. *Right there*—a very precise and contained place. After the baby's arrival, I was sure, I would continue to be exactly the same person as ever—the same wife, daughter, friend, and, yes, lawyer. My map would simply have one additional thumbtack: *baby*.

And then Sophie arrived. She was no longer a hypothetical baby—she was real. Quickly, I realized I'd been a complete idiot. Sophie wasn't a thumbtack on the world map; Sophie *was* the map! And everything else—and I do mean everything else—became the thumbtacks. Marriage? San Luis Obispo. Sex? Ha! Des Moines, if I was lucky. Friends? Barstow. Career? Detroit. Exercise? Ah, luxury: Paris. Sleep? *Sorry, we've run out of thumbtacks.*

But in those first glorious months of Sophie's life, I wouldn't have had it any other way. Sophie was my world. Even after years of loving Brad so deeply, I had never experienced a love like this before. Right after Sophie was born, Brad and I mutually agreed that, in the event of a fire, there was no question whom we'd both rescue: Sophie. *No offense,* we both said. *None taken,* we both answered.

When I took Sophie to my mom's house, I sat in a chair, holding Sophie and staring into her sleeping face.

"Oh, Mom," I said, "I love every inch of her, every cell, every molecule. I love her hair, her nose, her soft lips. The way she smells. Oh, I just want to eat her up. I've never been so in love in all my life!" After a moment, I realized the silliness of verbalizing these obvious statements to my own mother, a woman with whom I now shared the Universal Truths of Motherhood. "Of course," I continued, a knowing smile on my face, "I'm sure you felt exactly the same way about me."

My own mother, without a moment's hesitation, answered, "No, honey. You're pretty over the top."

I took an extended maternity leave from work to spend every moment with my beautiful baby. I would come back, I assured the firm, when Sophie was six months old. I was certain that six months would feel like an eternity. And then, after my brief respite as a full-time mommy, I'd be back to my old self.

Of course, six months passed in the blink of an eye. And I wasn't back to my old self. I wasn't even in the same universe as my old self.

"I can't leave her," I blurted to Brad on the eve of my scheduled return to work.

But we were tens of thousands of dollars in debt from law school, and Brad's salary alone wasn't enough to cover student loans and living expenses.

"We'll get a great nanny," Brad suggested. "She'll be fine."

I was frustrated that he didn't understand. "She might be fine. But *I* want to be the one to care for her."

"What about working part-time?"

Oh, please. "No attorney has ever worked part-time at my firm. Ever. That's not an option."

"Well, then, it's a no-lose situation," Brad said. "Just write up a proposal with everything you'd want in a perfect world, and submit it. If they say no, you need to find another job. If they say yes, you've got exactly what you want. It never hurts to ask."

I couldn't argue with Brad's logic.

Just as Brad had suggested, I wrote up a ridiculous proposal, incorporating all the elements of my dream work situation—part-time hours, working from home, and full benefits—and then I sent the proposal to the managing partner of my firm. The very next day, I received word that my proposal had been summarily accepted. It was the first arrangement of its kind at my firm. I didn't know whether to jump for joy or dissolve into tears. *Yay?*

For the next six months, I worked from home and relieved the nanny multiple times per day to breastfeed and cuddle Sophie.

I'm not sure which came first, the chicken or the egg, but Sophie wasn't attached to stuffed animals or blankies; she was attached to me, literally and figuratively. When I tried to put her in a crib, stroller, or high chair, Sophie wailed to the point of hyperventilation, until I picked her up and snuggled her close.

When I finally decided to wean Sophie, after her first birthday, I gave her a sippy cup full of warm chocolate milk in lieu of my breast, just as the leading baby book had instructed, and she threw it angrily against the wall, seething. I was her woobie. There would be no substitutes.

Every night, Brad bounced Baby Sophie in his arms for an eternity to put her to sleep. When Sophie cried hysterically in her crib, not wanting to be left alone, Brad scooped her up and brought her into our bed. When I protested, telling Brad she needed to learn to soothe herself, he wouldn't hear of it.

"Whatever she's crying about, it's real to her" was his mantra. "Bears don't leave their cubs alone in a cave, crying hysterically, or else they'd get eaten. It's basic wilderness survival, honey. We don't leave our baby to cry."

Chapter 18

Two years after I had Sophie, getting pregnant again was as easy as falling off a log. I told the doctor at my very first appointment of the pregnancy, "Doc, this baby's as strong as an ox."

The sonogram revealed that the little ox inside my womb was a baby girl. A Baby Chloe to join Big Sister Sophie. Sophie and Chloe. Two sisters. Just like Sharon and Laura.

In a flash, I was four years old. I had gone number two in the bathroom, and there was no toilet paper. As any sane four-year-old would do in this situation, I simply used the nearby hand towel to wipe myself. And then, in another perfectly logical (and, I believed, polite) move, I neatly hung it back up on the towel rack.

Some time later, six-year-old Sharon marched me into the bathroom and, holding the poo-stained hand towel out toward me in disgust, demanded, "Did you do this?"

"No!" I lied, feigning indignation.

But Sharon wasn't fooled. "I know you did it."

What Sharon did next shaped our sisterhood our whole lives: She helped me dispose of the mortifying evidence. Rather than rat me out to our parents, she led me and the "poo towel" (as it has come to be known ever since) into the back yard, where, after glancing around to make sure no one was watching, she hurled it over the back fence and into the neighbor's yard.

Genius!

I never would have thought of that. And that's why I needed a big sister.

I have never forgotten how it felt when Sharon chose to be my accomplice in crime, rather than the Gestapo. Even though I didn't know the terminology at the time, I thought, in essence: *She's got my back.*

And now I was going to have two little poo-towel huckers of my own, God help me.

Brad and I were ecstatic to have another baby, of course, but the pregnancy itself was just a means to an end. This time around, the giddiness of first-time pregnancy was replaced by the drudgery of "been there, done that." Morning sickness was no longer the happy emblem of a successful pregnancy; it was just me puking my guts out.

One day well into the pregnancy, I was sitting on the cold tile floor of the bathroom, retching violently into the toilet. Brad stood in the doorway, and just as I paused briefly between heaves, tears streaming down my red, puffy face, he asked, "Hey, where are my brown shoes?" I looked up at him and gestured that I was just a little bit busy at the moment. So much for ginger-root tea and foot massages.

Another time, when I was eight months pregnant, I asked Brad to bring a week's worth of groceries in from my car because my back was hurting.

"Well, how'd you get the bags into the car in the first place?" Brad asked, implying that same method would work again on this end of the journey.

It wasn't a glorious time for the two of us.

Unlike the baby growing in my belly, Crazy Buster, by then age thirteen, clearly was not as strong as an ox. The fur on his face had turned gray, and he grunted when he walked. It had been many years since he had tried to prove his dominance over puppies and Rottweilers.

In June 2002, when I was six months pregnant, Buster began vomiting and couldn't stop. We took him in to the vet, only to learn that he had a massive and terminal tumor in his throat. It was time to put Buster down.

Mere weeks before, Brad alone had sat at the bedside of his uncle Roger, his father's brother, holding his hand as the doctors removed his life support. Brad had taken on this responsibility to spare his father from doing so, but that final moment when the life had passed out of Uncle Roger's body had haunted Brad.

When we learned of Buster's prognosis that day, Brad broke down. "I can't do it again—not this soon," he whispered, his voice strained.

I took Brad's hand in mine. "I'll stay with Buster, honey. I'll be there in his final moment of life. You can go outside to the waiting room."

Brad looked at me, unsure. He started to speak, but I cut him off. "Go on, Buddy," I assured him. "I can handle it." My voice communicated supreme confidence.

But when the doctor came into the room holding a syringe with a three-inch needle, my knees wobbled and I began to weep. I bolted into the waiting room, where Brad was sitting with his head in his hands. "Brad! I can't!"

And so it was Brad, yet again, who remained strong in order to spare a loved one from pain. Thanks to Brad, and not me, Buster had a warm and loving lap to nuzzle when he took his last breath.

Just as I had predicted, when Chloe arrived, she was a baby version of Hulk Hogan: She was almost nine pounds at birth, and immediately bursting at the seams with innate self-confidence. And, in addition to being hardy, she turned out to be the easiest baby on Earth. She did whatever we wanted her to, *when* we desired. When we ate dinner, we placed Chloe in her high chair and she sat calmly for as long as we liked, eating whatever we put in front of her (anything from mashed carrots to carnitas).

I said to Brad, "She's a dream baby."

But Brad wasn't fooled. "Nah," he said. "That one's a wolf in sheep's clothing. We're gonna have to keep an eye on her."

I thought he was a fool.

But then, as Chloe's second birthday came and went, it started to dawn on me that maybe Brad was onto something there.

"You not saying right!" Chloe shouted at me when I flubbed

Gaston's line from *Beauty and the Beast*. She knew every single line and inflection, and she had begun forcefully directing the rest of us to deliver Disney-worthy performances on a daily basis.

"You're bossy," I retorted, fed up with her single-minded pursuit of glory.

"I not bossy, Mommy," Chloe said. "I sassy."

That one made me laugh. Yes, she was definitely sassy.

But as I laughed, I also marveled: I was having a conversation with my two-year-old self.

Not too long after that, after Chloe had committed some toddler infraction, Brad admonished, "Say you're sorry, Chloe."

Chloe's little lips pursed with defiance, and after a moment to consider, she calmly stated, under her breath, "Lorry."

Brad was incredulous. "You said *lorry*, Chloe. I heard you." We exchanged looks of disbelief. "Now, say you're *sorry*."

Chloe again considered her options. And, God help me, this is the absolute truth: That child—that *toddler*—looked Brad in the eye and said, in an even tone, "Sarr-uh."

The full breadth of Chloe's wolf-in-sheep's-clothing essence, just as Brad had predicted in her infancy, was revealed at that moment, and we now exchanged terrified glances: Chloe was Crazy Buster reincarnated. Only this time, we couldn't get a full refund from an Irish baby trainer.

Chapter 19

Countdown to chemo: three days.

I pulled up a website displaying a mind-boggling array of wigs on my computer screen. I knew the girls would come looking over my shoulder within minutes, as they always did, and I wanted to take the sting out of my imminent baldness. Sure enough, two little chins were quickly resting on my shoulders.

"Whatcha doin', Mommy?" Chloe asked.

"Just looking at wigs."

"How come?" Sophie wanted to know. "Are you gonna wear a wig because of the cancer?"

"I was thinking about it. Do you two want to help me pick one?"

They were excited. That sounded fun, not scary!

"Well, pull up a chair," I laughed.

For the next several hours, the girls and I had a great time poring over pictures of every type of wig imaginable. Blue wigs, red wigs, long wigs, short wigs . . . it was like wig shopping with Dr. Seuss.

"Oh, Mommy, you should get that one," Chloe cooed. When she pointed, it was to a long, platinum blond wig. Barbie hair. Chloe wanted her mommy to have Barbie hair.

I giggled. "Oh, Coco. I don't think so."

"But you'd be so pretty, Mommy."

Just the thought of myself walking around like that made me belly-laugh. "Thank you, Cokie. I'll think about it."

"What about that one?" Sophie pointed. No surprise there: It looked just like my old hair—long, brown, and thick. That's my pragmatic Sophie.

Okay, I thought. *She needs a return to normalcy.*

The next day, Brad went with me to a wig store that catered exclusively to cancer patients. With lots of silliness and only a few tears, he watched me model every type of wig, from a Joan Jett–style number to a red-haired, flapper-esque bob. Finally, though, I settled on something in the style Sophie had suggested: long, brown, and thick.

Let the hair falling-out begin.

Countdown to chemo: two days. I lay on the operating table in my hospital gown, waiting for the installation of a port—a catheter permanently implanted for easy infusion of the chemo drugs—into my vascular system. Brad had not been allowed to come into the operating room, and I yearned like a new kindergartner for him to hold my hand. I stared at the harsh lights above me and thought, still in disbelief, *I have cancer?*

And then, yet again, the tears flowed. I turned my face away from the operating-room nurse standing next to me, trying to hide my embarrassing sniffling.

"It's okay to cry, honey," she said, as she dabbed my cheek with a tissue. "This is the perfect place to cry."

Chapter 20

I imagine my family in the shape of an isosceles triangle—the three points composed of the kids, Brad, and me. When we're running on all cylinders, thick lines connect all three points. But when the girls were little, as Brad and I juggled demanding work schedules and sleep deprivation, I could feel the line between the parental points becoming perforated—our family triangle was becoming a *V*.

When either Brad or I had any free time, we spent it as a family foursome, or as individuals (golf for Brad, exercise or sleep for me). We rarely went out as a couple, other than for work-related events. We still enjoyed each other's company, but we were exhausted, and getting a baby sitter was a hurdle. Sometimes, in the middle of an argument, I'd hold up my index and middle fingers in the shape of a *V*, silently reminding him of our family's fate if he failed to tread carefully. That didn't go over very well.

And though I probably looked like I had it all together on the outside, I was scattered and anxious much of the time. My part-time gig wasn't nearly as ideal as I'd hoped. The firm had grown more and more impatient with me, wondering when I'd snap out of it and come back to work on a full-time basis. Clients or partners always called me on my days off, usually as I was strolling through the park or zoo with the girls. I would wave my hands frantically at the girls to be quiet, lest the person on the other end of the line discover—*gasp!*—that I was with my kids and not sitting at my desk. On workdays, I had started going in to the office—managing clients, documents, and court filings from home had turned out to be impossible.

Every month, my billable hours increased slightly, inching closer and closer to full-time, and I started to feel less and less in control of my life. It wasn't what I wanted, but it was unavoidable. I had no choice, I thought.

By this time, I'd reached the conclusion that trying to resolve conflicts in the legal system was like trying to breathe underwater: not effective unless you're a shark. The guilt of leaving my kids to do something I didn't even enjoy, plus the stresses innate in practicing law, were eating me alive. Occasionally, I'd say to Brad, "I'm going to have a nervous breakdown." He thought I was exaggerating. But I wasn't.

In addition to my garden-variety stress dreams—dreams involving snakes, or sitting for a math test without having studied, or being pushed onstage in front of a large audience without knowing which character I was playing—I'd started having a disturbing recurring dream, too: I was in a public place, and I had to go to the bathroom.

Right away. I frantically entered a dirty public stall. I quickly closed and locked the stall door, pulled my pants down to my ankles, and sat down on the toilet to do my business. Then I looked up, and only then realized that one of the stall walls, which should have been metal, was actually made of clear glass. *Surprise!* I was sitting on a toilet, doing my thing, in a department store window. *I was the Macy's window display.*

And feeling stressed out wasn't even the whole picture; I had begun to feel a general sense of malaise, an undefined disappointment, in my life, too. When I was younger, I had always felt like I had a super-secret ingredient for an exclusive Laura recipe that I alone was concocting. But now it seemed my secret ingredient had morphed into Velveeta. If I was being honest with myself, I had not become everything I had hoped.

As soon as these thoughts flitted across my mind, I felt guilty for thinking them, and I pushed them away. *You have a wonderful husband and two beautiful children,* I would say to myself. *You make a great living. You work part-time. It's a good life.* It was self-indulgent to feel anything other than gratitude. I had everything in the world.

I tried to convince myself that, contrary to my girlhood fantasies, living a simple life—wife, mother, part-time attorney—was my true destiny. Not becoming the next Judy Garland. Not winning the stupid Academy Award. It was time to grow up, to face reality. *Dreams are for kids. I should appreciate my simple, happy life.* My left brain had my right brain in a headlock, and it squeezed and wrangled until Righty was silenced yet again.

I was missing a big piece of my puzzle, though—a piece that

didn't negate my love for my family but simply enriched me as a person. I felt underutilized. I had created the life I thought I *should* want, rather than the life I actually wanted. But back then, I couldn't articulate any of that. I just felt overwhelmed and unfulfilled in a vague, undefined way.

If I was at the park with the girls, I was thinking of the legal brief due to be filed in court the next day. If I was at work, I was homesick, wondering what the nanny was doing with my girls. On my way home from work, I would fly through the grocery store without a second to spare. And when I got home, just in time to relieve the nanny, the home marathon would start: make dinner, clean up after dinner, bathe the girls, read to the girls, put the girls to bed. Say hello to Brad. Maybe work for an hour or watch TV. Maybe have sex, maybe not. Go to sleep.

The only thing I could articulate to Brad about how I was feeling was that I didn't want to be an attorney anymore. He had stopped practicing law years earlier and was now working in the commercial real estate industry, and I wanted to change careers, too. But I couldn't see beyond my idea of wanting to *leave* the law to the much more important idea: *What did I want to do instead?* Conversations (and arguments) between Brad and me typically focused on the pluses and minuses of my legal career. He thought the flexibility and paycheck of working as a part-time lawyer couldn't be beat. He thought I was being a pansy-ass complainer and that I should suck it up. He didn't understand why I was so dissatisfied with the arrangement, and I couldn't explain it to him.

"You can't quit working," Brad reasoned. "We need your income.

If not law, you're gonna have to figure out something else. And I don't know how else you could make that kind of money working part-time."

"Well, at what point could we afford for me to just quit? How much would you have to be making?" I asked.

"It doesn't matter," Brad retorted. "I don't want to be solely responsible for our family income. If I made three million a year, I'd still want you to work, at least part-time."

I was speechless. And trapped.

After hearing me complain for months on end, Brad finally threw up his hands and said, "Stop complaining about it, then, and go find something else to do. I'm sick of hearing about it."

But I didn't. I hadn't come up with an action plan beyond *complaining* about what I was doing.

Brad started golfing with his friends every weekend. I was offended. *He should be spending time with the girls and me, dammit!* But Brad is not, and has never been, a man who can be cowed into doing what anyone else wants. Rather than cut back on his golf outings, he suggested that I, too, arrange to have more fun.

"Maybe you should get together with friends more often," he suggested, deflecting my complaints. "It might give you the opportunity to . . . relax?"

This was a revolutionary idea, considering that outings with my friends had fallen completely off my world map since the girls had come along. Brad and I had just moved into a new neighborhood, and there were lots of ladies down the street I was hoping to befriend.

I had an idea: *I'll start a bunco league.* And so it was that the legendary Bunco Girls were born.

Have you ever played bunco? If not, here's what you do: Once a month, you and eleven other women drink wine, gab, gossip, and guffaw. After a little while, you drink a little more wine, gab a bit more, and then you . . . Wait, what do you do next? Oh, yes, you roll three dice. And count how many times the right number, whatever that happens to be, is rolled. If you happen to roll the lucky number on all three dice, stand up and shout, "Bunco!" (Heads up: Within seconds, someone is going to bean you on the head with rearview mirror–style fuzzy dice).

When the dice rolling has ended, eat a brownie or perhaps a piece of mud pie as you find out whether you have exhibited sufficient prowess to win a bunco prize, which might be a scented candle or a casserole dish. (Or perhaps a penis-shaped lollipop—it just depends on the crowd.)

Since I formed the group, the Bunco Girls consisted of two factions: "Laura's old friends" and "Laura's new neighbors." Most Bunco Girls had young children and, like me, were frothing at the mouth to have some girl-style fun.

With each monthly bunco session, rolling dice became less and less central to our purpose. What we were actually doing was creating a safe haven, an indispensable support system, for each other, a place to admit when we were saturated with temper tantrums and whining (by both our husbands and our kids). We commiserated about diaper duty, nighttime feedings, discipline, and childcare. We exchanged recipe ideas, book recommendations, and all manner of phone numbers for plumbers, baby sitters, hairdressers, and massage therapists, and we laughed. As time went by, we supported each other during pregnancies, divorces, injuries, and illnesses. Sometimes we cried and the dice remained untouched on the table.

Each and every time I returned home from bunco, I was surprised and relieved to see that Brad had capably put the girls to bed and the house was still standing. Not once did I come home to find my family huddling and shaking in a corner in their own feces, like dogs at the pound. *Not once!*

Now that we felt confident our husbands and children could manage—*briefly*—without us, the time had come for the Bunco Girls to venture out for a girls' weekend. In Las Vegas, no less. After kissing our husbands and kiddies goodbye, we piled into a limousine headed for the airport, wearing matching pink tank tops that read MOMS GONE WILD.

In Las Vegas, the Bunco Girls danced into the wee hours of the morning among the twentysomethings in the clubs. We lounged at the pool and drank fruity drinks with pineapple garnishes. We played blackjack and craps in the casino. We ate uninterrupted meals at fancy restaurants and resisted the urge to cut up anyone's meat but our own. We sat in the front row of the ABBA musical, *Mamma Mia!*, singing along to "Dancing Queen" and waving our arms in the air. We were like caged animals who'd been set free. And when we returned home, though our heads were pounding and our eyelids were drooping, we were revitalized and energized. We kissed and hugged our husbands and kids and thanked our lucky stars to have them. Our hearts were full.

She was up four times in the night with Baby

Can't think clearly to save her life

Laundry piling up is downright dreary

And the older one's begging for a pony ride

There's only one thing to do, if she wants to stay sane

She calls up her girlfriends all with babies on the brain

"Put your kids to bed, get your skinny jeans on

Bust me outta here, 'cuz I'm so far gone"

Moms gone wild, Mama needs a girls' night out

Moms gone wild, Lord knows she loves her child,

But Mama needs a girls' night out!

Chapter 21

Brad and his partner in crime, Sophie, had started making noise about wanting a puppy. Whenever we saw someone walking a Boston terrier along the sidewalk, they would coo, "Oooh, so cute!" and, "Let's get one!"

"A puppy would be good for the girls," Brad reasoned one day. "They would learn responsibility."

"No way," I said, without a hint of equivocation. Between work and the girls, I didn't have any extra energy or time to spend housebreaking and training a puppy. "I'm the one who's gonna have to take care of it, and I've got enough on my plate. Absolutely not."

"Oh, come on, honey," Brad tried to charm me. "It would be so fun to have a new puppy."

But I wouldn't budge. "No way."

"C'mon, honey," Brad persisted. He wasn't used to my resisting his charms.

"Brad, no." And, knowing my husband all too well, I added, "If you go out and get a puppy without my consent, so help you God, you will rue the day. Not only would you be the sole caregiver for that puppy—and how you would handle that while at work all day is beyond me—but you'd also have to learn to enjoy life with a wife who hates your guts."

I couldn't have been any clearer.

And so, a week later, right before a three-day weekend off from work, Brad and Sophie came home with a brand-new Boston terrier puppy—a little mound of fur that looked like a black-and-white guinea pig. He looked quite a bit like our poor, departed Crazy Buster, but even I could see that this one didn't have crazy eyes. He actually seemed pretty calm.

Still, I was livid. "I told you no!" I yelled at Brad. "*I told you no!*"

"I know," Brad soothed. "But isn't he cute?"

I was speechless.

Brad switched to a conciliatory tone. "Sophie and I went to a breeder just to look. And then the look on Sophie's face . . . I just couldn't say no."

Silent treatment. A volcano about to erupt.

"Buddy, I promise, I'll do *everything*," Brad coaxed.

"You got that right." I walked away in a huff.

Four-year-old Chloe, who had been just as surprised about this new development as I had, ran out into the alley behind our house and hollered at the top of her lungs, "We got a puppy!"—just as I had done thirty years earlier, when my parents (note to Brad: "my *parents*," plural) had brought Darrow home.

At Chloe's magic words, a horde of neighborhood kids descended upon the furball in Sophie's lap, oohing and ahhing and jockeying to hold him. The expression on Sophie's face was priceless—as if she had just sprouted magic wings that could fly her to Disneyland.

I wouldn't hold the puppy, cute as he was. And I refused to pet him. I knew we would wind up returning him to the breeder within mere days, and I didn't want to get attached. My heart ached for poor Sophie. She would be devastated when we told her the puppy had to go. She had just turned seven, and I knew she wouldn't be able to understand. But really, how could Brad have gone out and gotten a puppy against my express wishes? It was inexcusable. Irresponsible. Disrespectful!

Over the next few days, while the girls cuddled and snuggled the puppy, Brad became that dog's bitch. When I found a little puddle of puppy pee on the floor, I turned on my heel in the opposite direction, calling, "Brad!" When I found a little turd on the carpet, I just kept right on a-walkin', shouting, "Brad!" And Brad, bless his heart, was Johnny on the spot with the Nature's Miracle cleaner. At night, he woke up to take that puppy outside, and first thing in the morning, he did the same thing. He praised the puppy for every outdoor pee and poop, as if the dog had brokered world peace. Every day, Brad shoved the puppy blob through a doggie door over and over, just to show him how it worked. The dog looked quizzically at Brad with his Tootsie Roll eyes, as if to say, *I don't know why you keep shoving my butt through that little door, but I like it.*

"What should we name him?" Brad asked the girls enthusiastically.

I pulled him aside. "Brad, we can't name the dog. Once we name the dog, we have to keep the dog. And we're not keeping the dog. You see how much work it is, and you can't keep this up when you go back to work after the long weekend. And don't even *think* about me helping you."

Brad mumbled something that sounded a lot like, "You're probably right." He sounded dejected. It broke my heart, really, but our lives were complicated enough. We didn't need to take on another dependent being. This would teach Brad not to go against my explicit wishes. He needed to realize that, on occasion, I actually knew best.

The next day, as if on cue, the puppy flopped his guinea-pig body right through the doggie door all by himself and then trotted off outside to pee under a bush. The whole family, even me, cheered maniacally. "Good puppy! *Goooood puppy!*"

I had to admit, the puppy was a genius. And so darned cute. And sweet. I'd never seen such a calm, affectionate puppy before. He was already following simple commands, just out of an innate desire to please. It seemed that Brad and Sophie had picked out a truly one-in-a-million little dog.

Again, Brad asked the girls, "What should we name him? I was thinking maybe Boomer the Boston terrier. Or maybe Bruiser. Or Bubba?"

"No, Daddy," Sophie said. "Let's call him Buster."

Brad and I looked at each other. Although Sophie did not have any firsthand memories of our departed Crazy Buster, she had long been watching family home movies featuring her toddler self dressing Buster in socks and hats. But wasn't it weird to name successive dogs the same name? Wasn't it odd that George Foreman had, like, six sons all named George? Yes, we were pretty sure it was very strange.

"Maybe let's try another name?" Brad suggested. "How about Bandit?"

"No, Daddy." Sophie was certain. "He's Buster."

We shrugged. What's in a name? It certainly was easy to remember. I picked up the puppy and kissed his soft face. He was so warm. Just a little angel.

"Okay," I proclaimed. "He's Buster Francis Martín Hoffman Roppé II." And there was no chance anyone was going to return this sweet little puppy back from whence he had come.

A week later, I called Buster "Buzzy Wuzzy" when I

nuzzled his fuzzy face. And that's when I knew: I'd fallen hard.

You see, my name is Laura and I'm a hardcore nicknamer. It's a disease.

Buster the First was Buzzy Wuzzy, Buzz Saw, and Buzzard. And now Buster II would inherit all of those nicknames, and probably more.

Brad, my lucky love, gets to endure being called Bird and Buddy. Not too crazy, right?

Sophie, is Soph-a-Loph, Fifi, and Fee. Still within the realm of reasonableness, right?

But my little one, Chloe, is my nicknaming masterpiece, my magnum opus. She is Chlo-Chlo, Coco, Coco Chanel Number Five, and Coco Puff. Puff Daddy. She is Cokie, which morphed into Cokie

Roberts (a reference to the journalist) and Cokie Rabinowitz (a reference to no one). Cokie became Kookoo, which morphed into Kookoo for Coco Puffs, at which point I congratulated myself on artfully merging the Kookoo and Coco nickname branches.

You see? I can't stop.

When Chloe was about three, Brad and I became acquainted with another couple, whose son was on Sophie's T-ball team. After we'd been friendly with them for about six months, the husband told me he'd only just realized Chloe's real name.

"I couldn't figure it out," he said. "You never call her the same thing twice."

"Oh, you know how it goes with nicknames," I laughed. "What silly names do you call your kids?"

He looked at me blankly. "I call them by name," he answered. "By their given names." And though he didn't say it, I'm pretty sure what he meant to say was, "*Duh.*"

Chapter 22

Chemo Day had finally arrived. As Brad and I entered the chemo infusion room, I told myself I was She-Ra, Princess of Power. I was ready to rumble.

The chemo infusion center was a huge room with rows and rows of Barcaloungers, in which rows and rows of cancer patients—some better off than others—were receiving infusions from adjacent IV bags. Little whirs and beeps, as well as the sounds of televisions turned to low volume, filled the otherwise hushed room. My stomach was churning.

I smiled at the other patients as Brad and I walked to my Barcalounger at the end of the row. Some met my smile, but others, whose eyes were vacant, could not. They had been fighting this fight for a long time. I took a deep breath and settled into my chair, white-knuckled with fear. It was going to take about eight hours to administer my chemotherapy drugs, Nurse Julie advised me. The drugs had to be infused very slowly, or else severe complications—like a racing heart or closed throat—could occur.

Just do it already. The anticipation's killing me. I winced at my casual use of that particular idiom at a time like this.

Nurse Julie began slowly pushing a drug called Adriamycin—what the other patients called the Red Devil—into my port. It was blood red (hence the nickname) and was so toxic, I was warned, it would burn my skin severely if it were to leak during administration. The sight of it entering my body was horrifying to me.

After my first dose of Adriamycin had been administered, I visited the bathroom (wheeling my IV stand along with me) and was traumatized to see bright red, Kool Aid–colored pee coming out of me. Alarmed, I told the nurse about it.

"That's good," she told me. "That means the drug is going through you." She told me to drink tons of water to flush it through as quickly as possible.

Brad held my hand throughout the whole thing (except when I went into the bathroom). We talked. We stared at each other. We nibbled on bagels. He often touched my face or kissed my forehead.

The infusion itself wasn't too bad, actually. Exhausting, but not painful. But when I got home that night, a debilitating nausea descended upon me. I felt like I was dying. And, for the first time in my life, that didn't feel like a figure of speech.

A couple days later, hunched over and groaning in pain, I shuffled to the computer on my desk and wrote my first postchemo message to My Dearest Jane: "Oooh, Jane, I am having a rough go of this. Tried all the antinausea meds, but spent a grueling night. Slept with a bucket. Woke up today, and I can't eat, I am so nauseated. Brad is so sweet, he keeps making me protein shakes, but it's hard to get them down. I am going back to bed now, just wanted to ask for a cyber hug, and give you one in return."

Despite the time difference, Jane's reply came quickly: "Oh Laura, I am sending you massive cyber hugs. You can do this, you are a strong, beautiful, intelligent woman. You have the inner strength to get over this—even if your innards just feel like they wanna be your 'outtards' at the moment. I am holding your hand; I am sending you so much love. You can do this. We can do this!" Apparently, Jane had not encountered the same degree of nausea I had, though her chemo had, of course, kicked her butt, too.

For five days and nights after my first chemo, I lay in bed. Brad came in and out to check on me. The girls came in and out to kiss and hug me or tell me about their day at school. Even I came in and out of being there, so to speak, though my body was mercilessly there the whole time. But do you know who never left, who stayed by my side, even when I had deserted myself? Buster the Second. That sweet little dog lay in bed right next to me, nuzzling his body right up to mine, for five days and five nights. When I groaned in pain, he laid his head right on my chest, as if to listen for my heartbeat. When the house was quiet and everyone else was asleep, I looked into Buster's brown, buggy eyes, and I felt as if our souls were communicating.

Buzzy, you're healing me.

Love, he relayed back. He put his head on my chest and looked up at me with soulful eyes. He sighed.

A week passed, and, like magic, I emerged from the dark cave. I took Buster on a five-mile walk, gratefully breathing in the fresh air and sunshine. I played board games with Brad and the girls. I did laundry. And, I was thrilled to realize, I actually felt hungry. Just in time, because it was Turkey Day.

Brad and I took the girls up to the mountains for a big Thanksgiving feast with my entire extended family, who welcomed me with tearful hugs and heartfelt words. Dad in particular was beside himself with worry, telling me repeatedly how much he loved me.

I could not actually taste my favorite meal of the year, because chemo had dulled my taste buds (a common side effect). But no matter. This holiday was not about the meal.

After the dishes had been put away, I trudged into the kitchen, pulled out an electric razor, and announced to Brad and the girls and my entire extended clan of parents, siblings, aunts, uncles, cousins, nieces, and nephews, "Let's do this thang, people!" I knew my short hair wasn't long for this world, and I wanted to take control of the situation.

As I dragged a wooden chair from the dining room and seated myself ceremoniously in the middle of the kitchen, my large family assembled around me, tittering and laughing with nervous excitement.

"Okay, let's do it!" they responded back, readily understanding my need for a celebration—whether forced or not—instead of tears.

Through nervous giggles (and a few unavoidable tears), each and every family member took a turn swiping that electric razor across my head. And with each vibrating pass, I felt empowered. *You're firing me, hair? Oh, no—I quit!*

In short order, my hair was shorn to military standards, except for one solitary patch at the crown of my skull that looked like a tiny yarmulke.

Everyone in the family had taken a swipe—except for Sophie. She stood in the back of the room, alone, cowering, and unwilling to touch the razor. Slowly, the group's attention shifted to my sad little Sophie.

The room became hushed.

In a flash, the charade of our celebration came to an end. Sophie's anguished face brought us back to reality. This wasn't *fun*. This was ripping all of our hearts into little tiny bits.

"Sophie," one of her triplet cousins coaxed, "it's kinda fun." *Thank goodness for eight-year-olds.*

"You can do it, honey," I echoed, choking back tears. "C'mon." I wanted Sophie to feel more powerful than the cancer that had been stalking her mommy. I wanted Sophie to look back on this moment one day and remember that she had fought back.

The entire family added their words of encouragement.

Sophie timidly stepped forward, and Brad placed the buzzing razor in her slender hand.

Just behind me, I could feel the warmth of Sophie's breath on my cold, bare neck.

She hesitated.

"It's okay, honey," I reassured again from my chair in the middle of the kitchen. Hair shavings dusted my shoulders and surrounded my chair. The room had become quiet, except for the soft hum of the razor.

Sophie exhaled softly. Finally, I heard the razor rise up behind my head and graze the top of it oh so briefly—followed by a rising cheer from the family. It was hardly a swipe at all, more of a . . . touch. But still . . . Sophie did it.

After a pause, someone else relieved Sophie of the razor and she quickly retreated to the corner of the room again, but this time, she was surrounded by her doting cousins.

Someone else finished the job, leaving me with uniformly quarter-inch-long hair all over my head, just like Demi Moore in *G.I. Jane.* I was, once again, a badass.

On our way home from our Thanksgiving feast in the mountains, I ran in to the local grocery store to pick up a gallon of milk while Brad waited in the car with the kids. As I walked down the milk aisle, I passed a surly-looking dude—we're talking shaved head and neck tattoos—who winked at me and mumbled, "Hey" as we passed each other in the aisle.

Oh my god, I thought. *He thinks I'm edgy.* Little did he know, I had looked like a soccer mom in my not-too-long-ago past life.

Back in the car, I told Brad about my new boyfriend.

"You're hardcore," Brad teased.

"I'm a badass, honey. Didn't you know?" After all these years, how could he not know that about me?

But the interaction inspired serious thought a moment later. "You know what? I think I actually look better like this." I struggled to find the right words. "When I looked like everyone else and played by society's standards of beauty, I could never quite measure up. Now that I don't look conventional and I don't have the option to, I don't feel the pressure of conventional standards of beauty, either."

An entire lifetime of beauty magazines, hair highlights, and envying the perfect, preppy girls, and I'd wound up feeling best about myself when I was forced to abandon all the beauty aids. Go figure.

It was the first time I had glimpsed a new world on the other side of cancer. In the shower that night, I drew a smiley face in the steam that had accumulated on the Plexiglas shower door. Just for the heck of it.

Chapter 23

When Chloe was a preschooler, Brad and I joined a neighborhood coed softball team, perhaps in an effort to reinforce the spousal connecting line on our family triangle. At one of our games, a teammate complained that his legs were sore from having run a full marathon—just over twenty-six miles—a couple days earlier. That caught my attention for two reasons. First, this guy was not a paragon of athleticism. And second, I'd always wanted to run a marathon. It was on my checklist of things to do in my lifetime.

I turned to another softball teammate, a good friend named Mike, and whispered, "Well, if *he* can run a full marathon, then I most certainly can."

Mike replied, "If you do it, I'll do it with you."

That night, in true Mike fashion, he sent me a spreadsheet detailing our training schedule—exactly what mileage to run on exactly which days to ensure maximum preparedness on race day.

For the next twelve weeks, he and I trained together, per the exact specifications of his well-researched spreadsheet, running hither and yon around our neighborhood and talking nonstop about life, work, family, kids, religion, and music.

On weekdays, I would come home after a long morning run and shower and dress for work just as Brad and the girls were waking up. On weekends, Brad graciously took a rain check on golf to watch the girls while I did my longest run of the week.

I noticed that my waistline was slimming down and a spring had returned to my step. At work, my boss, Janice, wondered aloud why I was committed to this crazy goal.

"It seems so time-consuming," she observed. "Why are you doing this?"

"Because I promised."

"Who?" she asked.

"Myself."

By this time, Janice had fulfilled her dream of opening her own law firm, and I'd been working for her for the past few years. When she had first left our swanky firm several years before, I had just gotten pregnant with Sophie. "I can only do one major life change at a time," I had said, and had opted to stay behind at my original firm.

Right after Chloe was born, however, Janice had called me and asked, "Are you *ever* gonna come work for me?"

"I work part-time now," I'd warned.

"That's fine," Janice had responded. "You can work as much or as little as you want. I just want you."

And so I'd made the switch. My swanky law firm had grown tired of my part-time work schedule anyway, so it was perfect timing.

Several years into working at Janice's new firm, however, I had realized that I did not, in fact, share her dreams (though I'd duped her, and myself, into believing so all those years earlier).

"I guess I just lack ambition," I'd said to Janice recently, in an unguarded moment of self-reflection.

"Ha!" she had retorted. "I don't believe that for a minute."

And she was right. What I should have said was, "I guess I just lack ambition in the law."

But, I didn't say that. Either I hadn't admitted that truth to myself, or I was too spineless to say so to Janice. Regardless, it was clear to me that Janice and I were not cut from the same cloth when it came to the legal profession: Just watching how energized and excited she was, on a daily basis, about her law firm, about being a lawyer, and about acquiring new cases and clients made it painfully obvious to me how little those same things inspired me.

As time went by, Janice started pressuring me to work more and more hours; as it turned out, my part-time schedule wasn't working out so well for her, either. But I wasn't willing to forgo chaperoning field trips and after-school pickups—certainly not to spend even more time fighting over other people's money.

But rather than recognize, or act upon, the truth that lay in my heart, I opted instead to escape my doldrums and chase after my true self by running 26.2 miles. Logical, right?

Crossing the finish line of that marathon was a watershed moment. I had never felt so empowered in all my life. I had set out to do something "impossible," but with hard work and persistence (and certainly not innate athleticism), I had done it. I wondered what other "impossible" things I could accomplish by applying that same formula. I realized I'd been making excuses for years about why I couldn't pursue my most passionate self: *I can't because I have young kids . . . I can't because my job is too demanding . . .* I realized I'd stopped dreaming years ago, not because of any outside factors, but because I'd created imaginary electric fences all around myself. All at once, I looked around and those electric fences had ceased to exist.

The very afternoon after running the marathon, I sat down with my rubbery legs and a yellow legal pad, and I listed all the things I wanted to do before I died. Just one day earlier, that list would have included "run a marathon," but now I'd checked that item off the list. I scribbled down anything that filled my heart, without regard to *how* I could possibly achieve it or how silly it sounded.

I don't remember everything I wrote on my list that day. I know it included traveling to Australia (not yet done), and also writing a book (check!). But the entry at the tippy-top of the list, underlined and circled, was one word: *sing.* I wanted to sing. I didn't know how. Onstage? In a band? In a choir? On a street corner? I wasn't sure. But I knew, in my bones, I had to do it.

Tell me, baby, are you feeling scared, and
Do you wonder how you just got here
I'm hearing what you're saying and it sounds like you're blue
Uptown problems but they feel real to you
I love you, baby, but you're thinking too much

You're pushing me away and

I just wanna sing a love song, la la la la la la la la

I just wanna sing a love song, la la la la la la la la

Chapter 24

Back when I was eight, Mom's Magnum, P.I.,
look-alike boyfriend (a mustachioed heartthrob who also happened to
be a first-class mooch) asked me to sing him a song.

"Okay," I agreed, enjoying the attention.

As Magnum, P.I., leaned against our kitchen counter, spooning
an entire apple pie into his mouth, I sang Fleetwood Mac's "Dreams"
to him: "Now here you go again, you say you want your freedom . . . "
I drawled, expertly mimicking Stevie Nicks's lilting inflection and
slurred phrasing.

Magnum, P.I., spit out a mouthful of pie, he was so impressed.

"Hey now, girl. You can sing!"

The next day, much to my delight, Mr. Handsome came back
with a stack of record albums and song requests.

"'Don't It Make My Brown Eyes Blue,' by Crystal Gayle!" He
shoved a record album into my hands. "Oh, and how about 'Jolene,' by
Dolly Parton? That'd be a good one!" He pushed another album at me.

It was a defining moment: I could sing!

And now, all these years later, my inner child had been jogged loose, and she was furiously stomping her Buster Browns inside my head: *I can sing! I gotta sing!*

But where? How?

After much consideration—*should I audition for local community theater, go to karaoke bars, or maybe deliver singing telegrams?*—I decided what I wanted to do was sing in a rock band. (Not original, I know, but each time I said it out loud, it sounded less and less preposterous.) But how to achieve it? Rather than trying to build my own band from scratch, I figured my best bet was to find and join an existing, functioning band. Easier said than done. I was a thirty-five-year-old, married, minivan-driving mother of two. And if all that weren't enough, I was an attorney to boot. Not the prototypical front woman of a rock band.

What existing, functioning rock band would have me? I tried to visualize what that band would look like. First, and most obvious to me: They'd have to be all men. If this existing band already had a woman in it, then why would they need me? And anyway, I didn't want to poach on another woman's territory. Yes, definitely all men. Second, the womanless men in this band would need to be in their late thirties or forties, or, hell, even beyond, or else I didn't stand a chance. As a thirty-five-year-old woman, I'd be a Golden Girl to a group of twentysomethings. On the contrary, in a group of older men, I might still have a little game. Finally, these womanless, fortysomething-year-old men would need to play music I actually liked and wanted to sing: fun, recognizable cover tunes. But, truth be told, if numbers one and two were satisfied, I probably would have joined a polka band.

Now that I knew my criteria for the band of my dreams, it was time to find it. But how? Maybe there was a more professional, targeted approach than mine, but I simply followed my instincts: I went shopping online, the same way I'd have bought shoes on Zappos.com. But since Rock_Bands_Who_Let_You_Sing.com didn't exist, as far as I knew, I googled "San Diego cover band."

A handful of websites popped up. I clicked on the first link and was met with a band photo—four dudes and a feisty-looking woman. *Nope.* I clicked on the next link. Another woman. I clicked on the next link. A woman. *Dammit!* I clicked on the next link. Hey, no woman . . . *but these guys are toddlers.* I clicked on the next link. A polka band. Okay, my standards were a bit higher than I had thought.

The very last link on the screen was to a band called Cool Band Luke, a play on the classic movie *Cool Hand Luke,* starring Paul Newman. This was a good sign. Brad and I often quoted the movie's most iconic lines, such as "I can eat fifty eggs," "Just shakin' the stick, boss," and of course, "What we got here is . . . a failure to communicate."

I clicked on the link. Four handsome men stared back at me. Not a woman in sight! *Bingo.* I scrutinized their faces. It was hard to tell their ages from the grainy snapshot, but they were most definitely *not* in their twenties. *Bingo again.* I held my breath and clicked on a tab labeled "Song List." Up came a list of songs like "Mustang Sally" and "Brick House"—party standards. *Triple bingo!* I felt a tingling begin to course through my body.

After finding the band's email address, I composed a lengthy sales-pitch email, which I've abridged here to save myself too much humiliation (and you from boredom):

I am a 35-year-old woman who is looking to acquire backup vocalist experience. . . . I know some, even lots, of your song list. . . . [A]re you ever in need of a female backup singer or vocalist? I have no ego, I'd do backup and that's it, and you would not have to pay me. I just want the experience and the opportunity. . . . I am a local attorney. . . . You can see my picture on my firm's website, [website address], just to see that I am not a lunatic or something. . . . I know this is sort of random, and perhaps you will consider this bizarre, but I live by the philosophy that you never, ever "get" if you don't ask.

I read and reread the email, adjusted the phrasing to make it just right, and pressed the "send" button. I took a deep breath to control my excitement. *Calm down,* I told myself. *Really, you shouldn't get your hopes up. It could take days to hear back from them, if ever, and . . .*

Just then, I received an immediate email reply from a guy named Rob, the guitarist from Cool Band Luke: "Can you call me, please?" he wrote, along with a phone number. I immediately picked up the phone.

Rob and I hit it off. He had a dry, understated sense of humor and didn't take himself or the band too seriously. He was a straight shooter—not a cheeseball at all. I knew right away it was a fit.

"Your timing is incredible," Rob said. "The band was just talking today about maybe finding a female singer, trying to mix things up. There are so many classic female songs we'd love to play."

I was spazzing out. "Oh, great! Can I come to your next rehearsal and, you know, see if you guys like my voice?" Damn, my voice was sounding like a chipmunk's. *Get a hold of yourself, Laura!*

"Why don't you just send us your demo?" he suggested. "If we like what we hear, we'll arrange a time to meet in person and jam for a bit."

"Sounds great!" A little squeak escaped from my throat. *Laura, try to sound casual.* "Yeah, I'll just send you my demo." *Damn, now I was going into drill sergeant mode.*

We said our goodbyes and hung up. It was a great plan. Yes. I'd send them my demo, and if they liked it, we'd get together and "jam for a bit." *Awesome!* Only one little problem: *I didn't have a demo.* And telling them the truth was out of the question; I didn't want them to think I was an amateur (which, of course, I was). I would adopt the same attitude I always did: Fake it till you make it.

The next afternoon, Brad and the girls (by then ages six and three) came home from a daddy-daughter day to find me standing in the middle of our family room with a teenager whom I'd found online (after having googled "how do I make a demo?"). I was wearing big black earphones and singing my heart out into a fancy overhead microphone supplied by my new best friend.

"Hi, honey," Brad said tentatively. "Whatcha doin'?"

"Makin' a demo." I smiled. There was a pause as we stared at each other. *I'll tell you all about it later.*

And then, God bless him, Brad escorted the girls quietly out of the room.

I sent the guys from Cool Band Luke—Rob, Jann, and Buzz—my "demo" (pretending, of course, that I'd had it all along), and, after hearing it, they invited me to their next rehearsal! I was elated, but also nervous.

I showed up to Cool Band Luke's rehearsal at Buzz's house (with pizza and beer for the guys and flowers for Buzz's wife). I must have changed my shirt eight times in anticipation of our first meeting, trying to decide if I should show a little cleavage, or maybe go for "not trying too hard" in a T-shirt, or maybe just try to stay classy (as mandated by Will Ferrell's Ron Burgundy in *Anchorman*).

When I walked up the steps of Buzz's house in a semiclassy, flowery blouse that showed a tiny (but undeniable) peep of cleavage, I had butterflies in my stomach and my throat felt tight. But then I met the guys. These guys were funny. Patient. Talented. Family guys. *They were my people.*

In person, Rob was every bit as cool and easygoing as he'd been on the phone. And Jann, the bass player, who also managed the band's website, was warm and genuine. He echoed Rob's earlier amazement about my timing in contacting them.

"The band has been taking a break for almost a year," Jann said. "The day you emailed us was the very first day I had put the website back up."

It was fate!

And then there was Buzz, the lead singer, a big-hearted, frenetic bundle of creativity. Buzz picked up his guitar and began to play "Brick House." I took a deep breath and began to sing along to the music. The guys laughed at hearing a woman sing, "She's mighty

mighty, just lettin' it all hang out." When someone suggested we try Ike and Tina Turner's version of "Proud Mary," I squealed and told them how much I loved the song.

"If we do that one, I'll have to do the Tina Turner dance, like this," I proclaimed, jumping up and shaking my body around wildly like Tina Turner (though I probably looked more like Richard Simmons).

The guys clearly enjoyed that spectacle, but no one had made a definitive statement about whether I was in or out. And I couldn't get a read on how Buzz felt about my horning in on his lead-singer territory.

I decided to force the issue. "You know, I'd be thrilled to sing 'oohs' and 'ahhs' in the background, if that's what you guys want," I said, putting out a trial balloon.

"Nah," Buzz assured me. "I'll sing half the songs, and you sing the other half. My voice gets tired from singing all the time, anyway."

The other guys agreed unanimously. I was in!

We selected a crop of songs for me to sing, and then embarked on several weeks of rehearsals for our first gig together, at the upcoming county fair in Ramona, California: population 36,405. Every time I ran out the door, telling Brad I was going to "rehearse with the band" (usually followed by "Don't forget to give the girls a bath!"), I felt as if I'd been inhaling nitrous oxide. I was in a rock band!

On the day of our first "big" (but actually small) show, at the Ramona County Fair, I stepped onto that stage with *my band* and belted out songs like "Chain of Fools" and "Me and Bobby McGee," much to the thrill of my entire extended family (including Brad and the girls—who'd covered their hair with glitter for the occasion— Dad, and Sharon) and the Bunco Girls.

At first I couldn't hold the microphone steady because my hands were shaking so hard, so I just kept it in its stand. But once I'd made it through the first three or four songs, sheer terror gave way to unadulterated, childlike joy. I could barely enunciate the lyrics, my smile was so ridiculously wide.

The next morning, I still had that smile on my face, and I'd also acquired a grapefruit-size bruise on my right hip—the by-product of having banged my tambourine all night with an overabundance of enthusiasm and a deficit of technique.

I had reclaimed a part of me that had lain dormant for far too long. *I was me again.*

I was snowbound, homebound, rewound

Hellbound, desk-bound, headin' downtown

Dumbfound, round and round, racing like a Greyhound,

Lost and found, run aground, wearin' my crown

Looking for fun, just want a playground,

Nothing profound, won't check your background

Looking for fun, wanna be a hellhound

Let me expound, breakin' outta Jonestown

I'm free! Free! Free!

Got no fear in me, not scared to be me

Do or die, now or never

It's never, it's never too late

Shortly after my striking debut, Buzz bowed out of the band to pursue his original music. And just like that, I became the one and only lead singer of Cool Band Luke—proving once and for all that you can, indeed, shop for just about anything on the Internet.

With each performance after that, I learned more and more. For one thing, I figured out that singing in a rock band differed from singing in a stage musical, and that singing into a microphone was different from projecting my voice toward the back of a theater. For another thing, I began to understand the nuances of my voice—when it sounded good and when it sounded bloody awful.

Brad came to as many Cool Band Luke shows as he could. He was effusive in his praise when it was merited, and honest in his criticism, too.

"You're oversinging," he'd tell me, or, "You're making weird expressions with your face."

He was always right on the money. I soon realized, with Brad's help, that I didn't have to *sell* anything. If I trusted my voice, if I stayed in the moment of the song, then everything fell into place. I could stretch for notes or inflections that were outside my comfort zone; I just had to sing from my heart, instead of my head. *I just had to be real.* But, oh, wasn't that the lesson I'd been struggling with my entire life? Easier said than done.

Victor Borge, a comedian and entertainer, has famously said that laughter is the shortest distance between two people. But as I sang "I Want You to Want Me" for a room full of joyful people celebrating a wedding or a simple night out, I learned beyond a shadow of a doubt that *music* surely gives laughter a run for its money as a person-to-person expressway. At the end of a long night of performing, I'd often receive loving hugs and words of warm affection from partygoers—strangers—who'd come to feel an inexplicable, visceral connection to me, despite the fact that we had not exchanged a single spoken word all night. And it wasn't *what* I was singing that caused this reaction—God knows I wasn't charting any new musical territory. No, it was that, through music, our souls had danced together, even if our intellects had not yet been introduced.

My new vocation as the singer in a band made me a bit of a novelty at my day job. Several local newspapers and magazines interviewed me, and the resulting articles bore headlines like "The Verdict Is in: This Lawyer Can Sing" and "Lawyer Revels In Facing the Music." Attorney acquaintances approached me outside the courthouse to say, "Hey, I heard you've been singing in a band . . . "

I felt glamorous. I started to dress for work with a little more pizzazz. I bought a push-up bra from Victoria's Secret that created the illusion that my breasts (which had become woefully scrawny and misshapen from prolonged breastfeeding) were once again full and buoyant. When I walked across a crowded downtown street at lunchtime, wearing my push-up bra under my business suit, a guy in the crosswalk took a second look at me as I passed on by. I was Shelley Hack in the Charlie perfume ad from the '70s: *And they call her . . . Charlie!*

I felt like I had a secret life. I was an undercover rock star.

When I played a bar gig with the band one night, a drunk twentysomething guy approached me to ask for my phone number, unaware that my brawny husband was standing two feet away.

"I'm married," I responded, "to that guy." I motioned to my broad-shouldered, six-foot-four-inch husband.

"Oh, sorry, man," the guy remarked to Brad. "But your wife is hot."

That sentence seared my brain like an iron brand. *I was hot.*

Several months later, after considerable contemplation, I told Brad that I was thinking about restoring my droopy breasts to their prebreastfeeding glory days.

"I know this sounds crazy," I began, "but I've been thinking I might go in for a consultation about a boob job—"

Brad cut me off. "Great idea. I think you should."

That was a bit too enthusiastic. I paused. "I know it would be really expensive, but—"

"Aw, it's just money," Brad said. "We can always make more money. I think you should do it."

Wow. I wasn't expecting quite that level of immediate support. I paused again. "Well . . . I haven't made up my mind yet," I continued slowly, eyeing Brad suspiciously. "But I thought I'd just go learn more about it."

"I'm one hundred percent on board." There was another pause as we assessed each other for an instant. And then we both burst out laughing.

Brad always *had* been a boob man.

In addition to being a card-carrying boob man, though, Brad just wanted me to feel good about myself. A few months earlier, Brad's idiot friend had asked him why he "let" his wife sing in a band. Clearly, this guy didn't have a clue about Brad, or about me. Brad was ecstatic to see me performing, to see the light shining in my eyes. In fact, my newfound zest for life had made me sexier to him than ever before. And, as Brad and I both knew, Brad did not "let" me do anything, thank you very much; that wasn't how our relationship worked. But rather than explain all of that to his caveman friend, Brad simply said, "Happy wife, happy life."

Little did I know then that two years later, my surgeon would say, in a gee-whiz tone of voice, "You know, you wouldn't have felt that tiny lump if it weren't for your breast implant pushing it out and making it palpable. That implant probably saved your life."

A girl never loved her saline so much.

Thank you, boob job.

Chapter 25

In eleventh grade, I was sitting in my AP biology class, talking to my teacher, Miss Marrone, about what I wanted to be when I grew up.

"I think I'm gonna sing jingles," I said.

"What do you mean, 'sing jingles'?" Her tone was as if I'd said, "I think I'm gonna *scrape tongues.*"

"You know, like on a commercial," I replied enthusiastically. And then, by way of explanation, I sang, "Nobody does it like . . . Sara Lee!"

Miss Marrone didn't hesitate. "That's lame," she said matter-of-factly. "Why sing *jingles?* Why wouldn't you sing your own songs instead?"

Oh. I'd never thought of that.

And I pretty much never thought of it again . . . until twenty years later, when something inexplicable happened inside my brain.

I had decided to train for a second marathon. Why, I did not know. My dear friend and running partner, Mike, had briefly moved to the East Coast, so I'd be running this one on my own.

Before going out for a training run, I made a late-afternoon stop at the grocery store to pick up some produce for that night's salad. I was wearing running clothes, no makeup, and my long hair tied up in a knot. As I picked through the tomatoes in the produce section, the store employee stocking the adjacent celery said hello.

"Hello," I replied.

He looked me up and down from head to toe, and then said, "You're lookin' good."

I was speechless for a second. *Was that creepy, or not?* Had I done something to provoke that reaction? Not knowing what else to say, I just thanked him.

I left the produce department, still trying to decide what to make of it. *Was he . . . flirting with me? Or just being charitable to a thirtysomething-year-old woman dressed like a slob?* Whatever his motivation, I decided to make believe he was reacting to my undercover-rock-starness. And if that wasn't the reality, then I didn't want to know.

Fifteen years earlier, in my early twenties, as I'd jogged up a steep hill, a car full of teenage boys had come up from behind and had hollered at me, "You're lookin' fine!" But just as their car had come up even with me, so that the boys could finally see my front side, the catcalling had ceased instantly. One of the boys, sounding genuinely remorseful, had yelled, "Sorry, ma'am!" And then they had sped away.

I had stopped dead in my tracks, panting and sweaty, and had watched the car disappear up the hill. *Ma'am?*

And now here I was all these years later, recoiling from an un-solicited catcall at the grocery store. I couldn't have it both ways, I realized: Did I prefer to be "ma'am-ed" into humiliation or ogled into self-consciousness?

Ogled, definitely, I thought. *No question about it.*

After unloading the groceries at home, I hit the street for my run. I ran in silence, forgoing my iPod in favor of the rhythmic sounds of my feet striking the pavement. *Boom, boom, boom, boom.* The rhythm helped me think. Or, rather, it helped me *not* think. *Boom, boom, boom, boom. Damn, I forgot to buy parmesan cheese at the grocery store. Boom, boom, boom, boom. What on earth should I do for Brad's birthday? Boom, boom, boom, boom.* Now my mind began to quiet down. *Boom, boom, boom, boom.* I was going into a runner's trance. *Boom, boom, boom, boom.* And then, without warning, a melody began to unfurl in my head. *Fly, fly, fly.* The melody was crystal clear. *Fly, fly, fly.* That melody wouldn't leave my head. *Fly, fly, fly.* Yes, I was definitely hearing a song. *My wings will take me there . . . If I lie to myself, will you come with me? Make me believe you care.* Just like that, a full-blown song started pouring into my brain.

When I came home from the run, I raced upstairs to record what I was hearing in my head onto a digital recorder. Then I careened back downstairs and dive-bombed Brad on the couch.

"Brad!" I blurted, almost hyperventilating. "Listen to this song!" I sang him the entire thing from beginning to end: "There was a man at the grocery store today who told me I look good . . . " It flowed out of me as if I'd heard it on the radio a thousand times. "Is that a real song, or did I just make that up?" I asked.

"I've never heard that song before," Brad answered. "I think you made it up."

"I thought so. It's just that . . . I hear it so clearly in my head. Like it's a *real song.*"

Brad said he loved it. "One suggestion, though," he offered. "A grocery store isn't very cool. You should change the very first line to "a man in a *record* store." And thus my first song was born:

There was a man in the record store today
  who told me I look good
I was wearing angel wings and flower charms,
  and he said he understood
I told him I'd fly to the mountaintop,
  if my wings would take me there
I was wearing pretty lies to make me feel good,
  and totally unaware
Fly, fly, fly! My wings will take me there
If I lie to myself, will you come with me?
Make me believe you care

After that, the floodgates opened. By the time I stood lacing up my shoes at the starting line of the San Diego Rock 'n' Roll Marathon in June 2007, an entire album of songs had been bouncing around in my head for months. Songs came to me during training runs, in the shower, in the car, and in my dreams—basically all the time.

When I crossed the finish line of the marathon, I looked down at my watch: four hours, zero minutes, and . . . eight seconds. *Eight seconds?!* My goal had been to finish the race in fewer than four hours! My knees gave way and I started to feel woozy. I would have collapsed on the ground were it not for a fellow runner, who had grabbed my arm.

That night, I went to bed exhausted (and pissed I hadn't achieved my target time in the race). But in the morning, the achievement of merely finishing a marathon had worked its inspirational magic on my brain yet again, and my frustration had been supplanted by an unrelenting thought: *The songs in my head need to come to life.*

Chapter 26

The songs in my head were beginning to bore holes in my brain, but I didn't know how to get them out. Arranging the songs with Cool Band Luke wasn't an option; the guys didn't have the time or interest to launch an originals band. Brad suggested I find an existing originals band and see if they might be willing to add my songs to their repertoire. That sounded like a plausible idea.

I went online and found a band of fortysomething guys who had advertised on Craigslist for a female lead singer. I showed up at one of their rehearsals (and was relieved to confirm that "looking for a female lead singer" wasn't code on Craigslist for "looking for a prostitute"), sang the Pretenders song they had asked me to learn, and got the gig.

I rehearsed weekly with them for a few months, and ultimately debuted as their new lead singer at a couple of bar gigs. Only then, after we'd gotten to know each other a bit, and after I'd proven my work ethic and willingness to be a team player, did I tell them I'd written a bunch of songs.

"Maybe you guys would be willing to do a few of my songs along with yours?" I asked hopefully.

Several of the guys in the band seemed receptive to the idea. But the leader—and the band's sole songwriter—couldn't have been more prickly.

"Look, Laura," he said stiffly. "I write the songs for this band. And that's the way it's gonna stay. You just stick with singing."

I was grateful for his candor.

But if I was going to sing songs written by others, I realized, I much preferred singing the songs of Aretha Franklin, Prince, and Janis Joplin to the songs written by *that guy*. And, of course, though the musicians in the band were sweet guys, there was just no comparing the chemistry I shared with my Cool Band Luke brothers. I quit the band the next day, and soon learned (in an email their bass player sent to me inadvertently) that my departure had presented a golden opportunity for them to find a "younger" replacement.

I didn't blame them, though—my heart had never been in it.

The year was drawing to a close, and I still had not formulated a plan to produce the songs in my head, which I feared would drive me mad. I couldn't turn them off, and I couldn't get them out.

On Christmas Eve 2007, I attended a family party Sharon hosted. The whole extended family was there in full force—aunts, uncles, cousins, parents—including my beloved cousin Matthew, who is ten years my junior. Matthew is a brilliant musician, composer, singer, and songwriter, as well as a free-spirited, sensitive soul who cares deeply about the people in his life and of the planet at large. He is humble, sensitive, generous, and authentic. And a bit of an iconoclast.

Since age eighteen, Matthew has been recording albums and touring the world with his rock band, Rx Bandits, amassing high praise from critics and diehard fans all over the world. He's worked his butt off to achieve the worldwide success that has come to him. Yeah, what I'm saying is, my cousin's a rock star. And not an undercover one, either.

Although Matthew is a decade younger than me, I look up to him as somewhat of a role model. I distinctly remember a family dinner when Matt was eighteen (which he did not attend) right after he had dropped out of college to go on tour with his then-budding band. Our grandfather (Grandpa Wayne-o), a John Wayne sort of man, stated at the dinner, with patriarchal authority, that Matthew was making the biggest mistake of his life, that he should stay in school.

"Music is a fine thing to pursue as a hobby," Grandpa Wayne-o declared, "but it's not something to pursue as a career."

At the time, I was a twenty-eight-year-old top-billing attorney at a respected law firm, and I kept my mouth shut. I did not say, "Grandpa Wayne-o, I disagree. I think it's a great opportunity; isn't now the perfect time in Matt's life to follow his dreams?" No, I didn't say any such thing. Instead, I quietly sipped my club soda with a twist of lime, and looked out the window of the fine-dining restaurant, feeling relieved that no one could ever say that I was making the worst mistake of *my* life. I would never run off to the circus—no sirree, not me.

But Matthew, quite unlike me, didn't care what anyone else thought. He knew exactly who he was and what he wanted to do with his life. He knew his calling, and wild horses couldn't have kept him from it. (By the way, a decade later, Grandpa Wayne-o was prouder of Matt's success than anyone and made a point of telling me, "Laura Jill, the most important thing in life is to enjoy what you do.")

On that night at my sister's Christmas party in 2007, I sat next to Matt, who by then had become a successful musician and rock star, and I told him enthusiastically about my newfound passion for songwriting.

"I can't get the songs out of my head," I lamented. "They're driving me insane."

"I can relate," Matthew laughed. He suggested I come up to his studio in Seal Beach (about an hour and a half north of San Diego) to record a demo of a song or two. I thought my head might explode from sheer excitement, just like that bald guy's head in *Scanners*.

About two weeks later, I found myself in Matt's garage studio, gazing into Matt's reassuring brown eyes and timidly singing, "Fly, fly, fly, my wings will take me there . . . " as Brad looked on, nodding his encouragement. It was contemporaneously exhilarating and nerve-wracking to sing my songs out loud for other people. I felt exposed.

I had expected support and encouragement, of course—this was not a tough crowd—but I had not anticipated the explosion of excitement and praise that came my way.

"Wow, Cuz, I had no idea," Matt enthused, surprised to see a whole new side of his tightly wound attorney cousin.

"Neither did I" was my honest reply.

Later that night, we recorded a demo of the song. Matt, musical genius that he is, played guitar, bass, and drums on the track, and then added harmonies to my lead vocals, just for good measure. It was a Herculean effort for one session. And yet when we finished up the song a few hours later, Matt took a deep breath and said, "Okay, Cuz, you want to do another one?"

And so it was that, on one of the most joyous nights of my entire life, two songs that had previously existed only in my head—"Fly, Fly, Fly" and "Girl Like This"—became audible in the real world. In a flash, I realized I'd been living in Dorothy's black-and-white Kansas for the past decade. But thanks to Matt, I waltzed right through the front door and into Technicolor Oz.

You've never seen a girl like this,
with magic in her fingertips,
Outside the lines, with eyes that shine . . . so bright
You've never seen a girl before, makes you walk,
no run, right through a door
A door you swore you'd never walk before . . . in life
You've never seen a girl sashay, with a way,
with a way to make you stay
Get down on your knees and pray . . . all night
You've never seen a girl like this . . .

On the drive home from Seal Beach, Brad and I listened gleefully, over and over again, to the two demos Matt and I had created that night. The recording process itself had been utterly thrilling for both of us, and each time we listened to the songs, we relived that rush again. But, in addition to experiencing the sensation of bringing my songs to life, Brad and I were blown away by the actual finished product. We weren't sure, and we knew we were biased, but . . . it seemed like these songs were pretty good.

"They're better than most of the songs I hear on the radio," Brad declared.

The next morning, when we played the songs for the girls, they were effusive with praise.

"Oh, Mommy! That is so good!" they squeaked.

And when I emailed the songs to Rob and Jann, my brothers in Cool Band Luke, they were over-the-top enthusiastic. Same thing with Dad and my good friend Pete at work. My confidence was building.

Finally, bunco night arrived and I played "Fly, Fly, Fly" for the Bunco Girls. Their reaction was as if I'd discovered a golden ticket in a Willy Wonka chocolate bar.

"You need to do this!" Bunco Girl Tiffanie commanded, as the others bum-rushed me with excited congratulations.

By the time I left bunco that night, my unrelenting desire had become an obsession. I was now a rabid dog, trotting down the street and frothing at the mouth: *Record . . . album . . . now!*

Chapter 27

Dear Laura,

Chemo! You get to feel the crappiest you've ever felt in your life, physically and emotionally; you look the absolute worst you've ever looked; and people pity you. And the best of all? You know it's all coming around again very soon. Happy days! Sorry, Laura. Whinge over.

Love Jane xx

My Dearest Jane,

If you think you could go through chemo and still have a recurrence or die, it is maddening. But if you just think that the chemo is the treatment to cure you, it makes all the difference. You take the medicine, and that's that. Disease. Cure. Done.

I am squeezing your hand, Jane.

XO Laura

p.s. What's a whinge?

Two weeks after my first chemo infusion,

it was time to get back on the horse. My cousin Matthew was in the midst of recording an album with his band, but for me, he traded a recording session for a chemo session. As the nurse led Brad, Matt, and me past the rows of cancer patients receiving infusions, all the way to my designated Barcalounger on the far end, Matt's eyes widened and his jaw clenched. As the bright red fluid entered my body through my port, a flurry of emotions flitted across his expressive face like a scrolling news ticker: fear . . . love . . . worry . . . anguish. Heartbreak.

The whirs and beeps of the chemo monitors and the scattered conversations of other patients filled the room. Matthew pulled out his acoustic guitar and began to play one of my songs, "Daddy's Little Angels," which he and I had composed together in my living room the night before. I was surprised to hear my own voice, unchanged and joyful as ever, emerging from my throat and singing the words to my song. As my body was anchored to the Barcalounger by a chemo IV, my soul flew around the chemo lounge, full of joy to be set free once again. For a moment, I forgot where I was, and that I was fighting to save my life.

When my eyelids began to feel heavy and flickered shut, Matthew quietly began singing Sam Cooke's "Wonderful World." His earnest voice was warm and comforting, like a fuzzy blanket. At the end of the song, the nurses and patients quietly applauded and asked for more. Music had proven itself to be the shortest distance between Matthew and every person in that room.

Back at home, I crawled into bed to await the inevitable post-infusion pain.

"Bye, Cuz," I whispered, as he leaned over to kiss me. "Matt, your music was such a gift today. And not just for me—for all the other patients, too. Thank you."

Matthew's big, soulful eyes were moist. "Cuz, I'm the one who received the gift today."

It didn't take long: I felt the nausea at my door within an hour, banging furiously like an angry beast, but the new antinausea meds Dr. Hampshire had prescribed me were a thick, bolted door keeping the monster out. Instead of the nausea this time around, I felt searing bone pain and can't-lift-my-head weakness.

Lions and tigers and bears, oh my. This was worse than the first time around.

Dr. Hampshire explained that the toxins from the first infusion had already settled into my system, and that with each subsequent infusion, my body tissue would become more and more overloaded. "With each chemo infusion," Dr. Hampshire warned, "it will get harder and harder."

All I could do was lie in bed with Buster by my side, not sleeping, yet not able to move, either. I was stranded in bed like poor James Caan in *Misery*. And chemotherapy was my ankle-breaking Kathy Bates. *My number-one fan.*

On the fourth day, Mom and Sharon came over to care for me. The three of us lay in bed together, just like the old days (except that in the old days, Mom's younger daughter wasn't listless and writhing in pain).

After our bit of nostalgic three-way bonding, Sharon got up and busied herself with my laundry while Mom went downstairs to make me scrambled eggs and dry toast.

"I can't eat it, Mom," I mumbled when Mom put the aromatic plate of food under my nose. "I'm so sick, Mom. I can't do it." Indeed, I felt as if my body were made of lifeless cardboard.

"You have to eat, sweetie," Mom coaxed. Tears were in her eyes. "*I need you to get better.*"

I was about to console her, when she added, "If you don't get better, who's going to take care of me in my old age?"

There was an awkward silence for a moment as I tried to decide if Mom was joking or not. Finally I mumbled, "Wow, Mom. For some reason, that just doesn't motivate me."

Mom burst out laughing. As usual.

Suddenly, I was back in her Honda, learning to drive a stick shift at age fifteen. I was in the driver's seat at a red light, as she reminded me what to do when the light turned green.

Yeah, yeah, I know, I told her.

But when the light turned green, I stalled the car. And I could not get that car to move. Cars behind us started to honk vigorously as the light went from green to yellow and back to red. I became frantic amid the din of angry horns.

And what was Mom doing this whole time? Laughing. So hard that tears ran down her face. She could have yelled at me, or demanded to switch seats so she could get us out of there in a jiffy. But no, she just enjoyed the ride, stalled though it was.

And now here she was, spooning scrambled eggs into her ailing daughter's mouth—trying desperately to enjoy the stalled ride. The strain on her face told me she wasn't succeeding.

A few days later, my hair fell out, just as Dr. Hampshire had predicted. When I brushed my teeth, little hairs fell into the sink. When I showered, hairs covered the drain. When I woke up, hairs dusted my pillowcase.

Jane and I wrote to each other almost daily to track the "progress" of our hair loss:

"I am a mangy dog."

"More hairs on the pillowcase this morning."

"Each shower is a fantastical journey of hair loss."

"Scratched my head and six hairs came out."

"Brushed it and the hairbrush was full."

"I am a Gregorian monk."

"I am Squidward in *SpongeBob SquarePants.*"

"I am one of the ESP triplets in the goo in *Minority Report.*"

Brad had been getting a kick out of rubbing my shaved head like a good-luck charm, but now I had to tell him to stop. My scalp hurt too much. Instead, I came up with a new game for him to play:

"Brad, come here," I beckoned. "Pinch some of my hairs."

Brad gamely pinched a lock of my short hair with his index finger and thumb, and then gasped as the hairs came out of my scalp like a knife pulled from warm butter.

It was oddly addictive. "Can I do it again?" he asked. "That's kinda fun."

"Knock yourself out, babe."

Chapter 28

Having a dream didn't mean I knew how to make it a reality. Producing an album with my cousin Matthew simply wasn't an option. He was touring almost constantly with his band; plus, he had several side projects that consumed his spare time. And I didn't want to rely on anyone's goodwill, anyway. It was imperative to get this thing done right now. I was consumed with an inexplicable sense of life-or-death urgency: I had to record an album before it was too late.

My online research revealed that there were countless professional recording studios and producers to choose from in San Diego and beyond. How would I be able to discern the "real deal" producers from the poseurs and con artists? It was intimidating. I called several studios and talked to their resident producers. Mostly they were nice enough, and clearly knowledgeable about music and recording, but my gut instinct told me to move on. Then I saw that one of the local studios boasted a Grammy-nominated producer named Steve Wetherbee. That certainly caught my attention, so I called and spoke with Steve for about half an hour. I was impressed by his obvious love of music, and also by his warmth and sincerity. When he invited me to come down to his studio to talk in person, I didn't hesitate.

Walking into Steve's studio felt like entering a church. It was the kind of studio you see in music videos, where the producer sits at a massive control panel riddled with countless levers and buttons while, on the other side of a Plexiglas wall, a recording artist sings into a grapefruit-size microphone.

This is where the magic happens, I thought.

I played my two demos for Steve, and he complimented my voice and songwriting, as well as Matt's musicianship.

"Do you have any more demos?" Steve asked.

"No," I told him. "The rest of the songs are in my head."

"How many additional songs are we talking about here?"

"Maybe . . . ten?" I answered.

Steve seemed intrigued. "Will you sing them for me?"

Pushing my nerves aside, I sat down on a stool and proceeded to sing every one of the songs that had been bouncing around in my head for months. After each song, I offered details I had imagined: "On this one," I explained, "I hear a violin line like *this,*" and then I hummed. "And on this one," I continued, "I'm thinking sort of a Bonnie Raitt feel, with a guitar riff sort of like *this.*"

Steve said my songs were catchy and memorable and my voice was unique. And, he added, the song structures were really strong—quite surprising for a neophyte songwriter. "You should make an album of these songs."

No kidding. Or else I'm going to lose my mind.

Steve said he could produce and record the album at his studio, including enlisting all the studio musicians I would need. But, of course, all of this was going to be expensive—akin to buying an economy car.

Small price to pay, I thought.

When I got home and told Brad about it, he said it sounded really exciting. But when I mentioned the price tag, he laughed out loud and said it was out of the question.

"But, honey, Steve says my songs are really good," I argued.

"Of course he does, babe—it's like the Barbizon School of Modeling: Anyone at all can go in there and be told, 'Oh, yes, you should be a model,' as long as they pay the modeling-school fee. That guy would tell anyone with enough cash that their songs are good."

I was speechless. And deflated. *My songs* are *good,* I said to myself. But, it seemed, that was that. This wasn't the kind of purchase I could make without Brad's consent, just as I wouldn't expect him to go out and buy a car (or a puppy, for that matter) without consulting me.

No matter how hard I tried, though, I couldn't let it go. My determination only escalated with each passing day.

The next week, Brad and I were preparing for an upcoming family ski trip to Utah for Presidents' Day 2008. As we packed, I could barely think about what gear the girls would need for the slopes; my thoughts kept drifting to the album I was increasingly desperate to make.

"Brad, can I get a new car?" I asked, as he stuffed ski pants and goggles into a duffel bag. For quite some time, he had been suggesting that I drive something more fun than my minivan.

"Yes, absolutely," he answered.

"Thanks, but I'd rather have an album."

Brad rolled his eyes. I had tricked him. "Honey, why are you so focused on this? Why can't you just record some more demos with Matt now and again, whenever he's back from tour? Why do you have to go so . . . *big* with this?"

I surprised myself by starting to cry. "I don't know," I answered honestly. "I just feel this life-or-death urgency about it. Like, I *have* to do this *right now.*" I was sobbing now. "I don't want to die without doing this, babe. I don't want to lie on my deathbed and realize my kids don't know who their mommy is!" I was a blubbering mess.

Brad was confused by my sudden outpouring of fierce emotion. "Okay, honey, but why do you have to produce the album at such a professional level? If it's just a vanity project, just a legacy to leave to the girls, then you don't need anything more than demo quality."

I was so frustrated! I could barely speak. "It has to be the absolute best quality I can manage. It can't be demo quality. I can't explain why. I don't know why."

Brad wasn't on board. And I was incapable of explaining this ferocious need I felt all the way down in my bone marrow. We were at an impasse.

The next morning, we piled into the car for our nine-hour road trip to Utah. While the girls happily watched *Shrek* on a portable DVD player in the back seat, Brad and I reveled in spending hours of unfettered time together. Between the girls, work, and the daily goings-on of our busy life, we hadn't spent this much undistracted time together in as long as I could remember.

We listened to music for a while, watching the desert landscape whiz by. The girls had fallen asleep in the back seat.

"Sing me your songs," Brad suggested.

I was overjoyed. Up until that moment, he had caught only snippets of the songs in my "collection"; he had never heard each one from beginning to end.

I sang my heart out for Brad, and then explained in excited detail the way I envisioned arranging each song.

"On this one," I told him, "I want the bridge to come way down, sort of like this song," and then I played a John Mayer song on my iPod. "And on this one, I want the feel to sound something like this," and then I played him an Alanis Morissette song. As I shared these thoughts and feelings with Brad, relief and joy spread through my body. Now he could hear what had been plaguing me for so long. Now he could finally understand.

Brad seemed stunned. "Wow, those are really, really good, honey. I had no idea."

I beamed at him. "You think so?"

"I do. Maybe I should at least talk to this Steve guy when we get home."

I nodded. That sounded like a plan. In truth, I thought my heart would leap out of my chest like that squid monster in *Alien*, I was so overjoyed at this concession. But for the time being, I tried to push the album out of my mind and focus on our family vacation.

It wasn't hard to do: The girls were endlessly entertaining on the slopes. Sophie snowplowed down the mountain methodically and cautiously, while Chloe careened down like Evel Knievel, oftentimes duplicating the "agony of defeat" fall from ABC's *Wide World of Sports.*

At the end of the week, as we made the long drive home from Utah, I looked over at Brad. He seemed in high spirits, despite having just received a speeding ticket from a pleasant policeman named Officer Malcolm. My heart bubbled over with love for my husband. I turned around to peek at the girls, sleeping sweetly in the back seat, and thought how young and innocent they were. They had so much life ahead of them, and they knew so little about the important things. I was overcome by an all-encompassing love for my family.

In a flash, my thoughts turned to worry. *What if my girls had to grow up without me?* I thought, shuddering. *What if I had only five minutes left in this world to tell them everything they'd need to know to grow up right?* I searched the car frenetically for a scrap of paper. And within twenty minutes, I had scratched out all the words and melody for a song called "Little Daughter."

When I had finished writing, I turned to Brad. "Listen to this new song, honey."

Tears sprang into Brad's eyes from the first moment I began singing, and they kept coming until the last line of the song. When I had finished, he wiped away the tears and cleared his throat. "Babe, that is beautiful," he said softly. And then, to my amazement, he added three little words that sent an electric current shooting through my veins: "Let's do it."

Chapter 29

When we got home from our family ski vacation, Brad and I visited Steve, the producer I'd been lobbying to hire, at his impressive studio. An hour later, as Brad and I settled back into our car, he conceded, "It's not the Barbizon School of Modeling after all."

A few weeks later, I was happily embroiled in the time-consuming (but thoroughly enjoyable) task of recording a full-length album. Up until then, I had thought a song was recorded when a band of musicians simultaneously played their instruments, all together, in a studio. As I found out through working with Steve, however, although that may have been how records were created in the "olden days," it was not how modern records were usually recorded.

In the modern era of music production, a song is typically constructed methodically, one track at a time. In the case of my songs, we recorded my "scratch" vocals (a rough draft of my vocals, to be rerecorded later) accompanied by an acoustic guitar played to a "click" (a computerized beat, erased later, that ensures the tempo of the song stayed steady throughout). Next, using the scratch vocal–acoustic guitar track as a blueprint, musicians recorded a rhythm bed—rhythm guitar, bass, and drums—that formed the foundational structure, the "bones," of each song. Only when we had recorded the rhythm tracks for all twelve songs on the album did we begin to add the instruments that would give each song flesh for the bones. Over the next several weeks, a steady stream of professional musicians came in to add lead guitar, banjo, mandolin, violin/fiddle, keys, and percussion. Even Matthew came to the studio to record guitar on several tracks.

Throughout almost all of the recording process, Brad sat in the studio with me, soaking it all in and grinning from ear to ear. On many days, Dad showed up, too, equally excited to watch the songs come to life.

Many years earlier, when I was seven months pregnant with Sophie, Dad had hired me as his lawyer in a business dispute. It was a small case, but Dad had wanted to fight it on principle. And anyway, it was a chance for him to hire his pregnant attorney daughter. And that was a hoot.

I called the opposing attorney, an old-school guy who thought attorneys had to yell to make a point, and suggested we meet in person to settle the case. The attorney's tone was instantly belligerent as he doggedly demanded that Dad and I drive to his Los Angeles office for any such meeting.

"We're gonna do this my way," he blustered.

"I'm seven months pregnant," I replied evenly. "I can't sit comfortably in the car for a two-hour drive."

What could he say to that? A few days later, in my San Diego office, Dad and I sat, composed, at one end of a marble conference table while the opposing attorney and his equally cranky client sat, red-faced and agitated, on the other end. Their arms were crossed.

At my opening settlement offer, the other client banged his fist on the table and shouted that we were wasting his time.

With the faintest suggestion of a swoon, I held one hand up in the air and my other hand on my swollen belly. "I simply cannot be subjected to this vitriol," I declared delicately. And to the attorney, I said, "We'll step outside while you get your client under control." With that, I marched out of the conference room belly first, with Dad trailing dutifully behind me.

After Dad and I had made our way down the hall, into another room, and had safely closed the door, we dissolved into laughter.

"This is so much fun," Dad said, and hugged me.

And now, sitting in Steve's studio, soaking up every moment of this wild ride, Dad's elated face made it clear: He was just as proud of his singer-songwriter-dream-chasing-sword-swallowing daughter as, if not more so than, he'd ever been of his fast-talking-attorney daughter. It was an epiphany for me: Dad didn't care if I was a lawyer, a singer, or the sword-swallowing bearded lady; he just wanted me to find passion and be happy. All those years of trying to garner his approval in a "respected" profession, and—I'll be damned!—he was a card-carrying member of the Laura-the-Dreamer Fan Club. He just . . . loved me.

Once all the instruments had been recorded, it was time for me to record my vocals. There was a steep learning curve to singing in a studio, as opposed to onstage, I learned, but Steve was very patient with his inexperienced recording artist. When I sang with my live band, my voice competed with so many other sounds that an off note wasn't fatal. But on a studio recording, every nuance and quirk in my voice was laid bare for all to hear. Singing for a recording, I soon figured out, required the utmost subtlety—something that had never been my strong suit.

It was right then in the recording process that a girlfriend of mine emailed me to tell me about a music contest put on by country superstar Kenny Chesney. Chesney was working with radio stations across the country to find the Next Big Star who would open for him at his arena concerts. All a person had to do to enter the contest was submit a recording of his/her original song.

"You should enter one of your songs!" my friend wrote to me.

I decided to submit my song "Mama Needs a Girls' Night Out," a decidedly country ditty, but we didn't have the background vocals recorded yet. The deadline for submission to the contest was fast approaching, so we had to move fast.

Steve was game, and came up with a great idea for a sing-along feel to the song.

"Can you get a group of your friends here this Saturday to record background vocals?" he asked.

Does Dorothy wear gingham?

On a sunny Saturday afternoon in late April 2008, the Bunco Girls crowded into the recording studio, thrilled to serve as the (country-flavored) Pips to my Gladys Knight. It was a case of life imitating art, or maybe the other way around. As Steve checked the microphones and set the sound levels, the Girls guzzled champagne, giggling and hooting like bridesmaids at a bachelorette party.

When it was finally time to record their vocals, the Girls snapped pictures of one another and shrieked with glee as they put on their fancy studio earphones. It was like herding cats, they were so amped up.

Finally, the group sang together: "Moms gone wild! Mama needs a girls' night out!" Their faces were a picture of unadulterated joy. As Steve and I watched them from the producer's booth on the other side of the Plexiglas, we couldn't help but laugh out loud.

When Steve turned his head away at one point to adjust a dial, one of the Girls quickly lifted up her shirt and flashed me, causing me to scream in shock and clamp my hand over my mouth.

Steve snapped his head up, not having a clue about what had just happened, and looked around. "What'd I miss?" he wanted to know.

I just shook my head and laughed.

Some of the Bunco Girls could sing pretty well, actually, while others were completely tone deaf. But vocal chops were not necessary to sing along to this particular song. Only exuberant energy and a soul connection to the song were required. And these girls had both, many times over.

Within a couple of days, Steve had expertly integrated the Bunco Girls' voices into the song, and I submitted it to the Kenny Chesney contest. The top four finalists would be chosen after one week of online voting by the radio station's listeners. For that week, word spread like wildfire among my friends, and their friends, and theirs, that a local mom/attorney had entered this big contest. When I picked the girls up from school, fellow moms shouted to me, "I voted for you!" and flashed me a thumbs up. Every time I checked the radio station's website that week (which probably amounted to over four thousand times), I was clobbering the competition. I couldn't sleep a wink at night from the excitement, and yet I wasn't the least bit tired by day. In fact, I felt thoroughly energized.

At the end of the week, Brad, the girls, and I huddled around our radio, awaiting the results of the contest, scheduled to be divulged on the morning show. And then we heard it. There was my voice, belting out "Mama Needs a Girls' Night Out," on the radio: "She was up four times in the night with Baby . . . "

Winning the Academy Award could not have felt any better than hearing my song on the radio for the first time.

"Wow, I bet lots of women out there can sure relate to that one," the DJ said. And then she went on to play the three other finalists' songs, leaving Brad, the girls, and me to jump for joy in our family room.

Shortly after that, there was a rap at my back door. My neighbor Bunco Girl Tiffanie was standing there with a huge grin on her face.

"I just heard your song on the radio!" she shouted, and she joined our family jump-fest.

A few minutes later, the radio station called to officially confirm I'd been selected as one of the top four finalists.

Awesome!

Even more exciting, the contest organizer told me, two weeks from then I would battle for the win against the three other finalists in a live "battle of the bands" at the San Diego Hard Rock Cafe.

Double awesome! . . . Wait, what? Only then did it dawn on me: I didn't have a band.

Chapter 30

Don't panic, Laura, I thought. I had a couple of options here. First, since the studio musicians on the record already knew all of my songs, the most pragmatic thing to do was to hire them to play the four-song set at the Battle of the Bands. *Simple.* But after a round of phone calls, I was crestfallen to find out that every single one of them was already booked for the night of the contest, a mere two weeks later. Not yet panicked, I went with option two: I called the guys from Cool Band Luke. Jann, my bass player, was unequivocally in. *See? It's all gonna work out.* So was my drummer. *Another relief.* Rob, in his characteristically self-deprecating fashion, said he'd play guitar for me, too, but he thought I should get a professional if I could. I assessed the situation: I needed a violinist, a keyboardist, and possibly a guitarist. *No biggie.*

I did what I always do when I need to locate a difficult-to-find item: I shopped online. A website catering to bands and musicians led me to a photograph of a beautiful blond woman with a violin. The music samples on her website varied from classical to bluegrass. *Bingo.* When I called this violinist, Jennifer Argenti, we clicked. She was soft-spoken and sweet, an absolute doll, but she was more than that, too: She had played in the Santa Monica Symphony for years, as well as with numerous rock and country bands. Several years earlier, Jennifer had left a corporate career to pursue her music full-time. On top of all that, she was the Western Surfing Association's Women's Shortboard West Coast Champion of 2007. My kind of woman.

Jennifer said she'd love to play with me at the Battle of the Bands. "Do you need any other musicians?" she asked.

"Well, actually, I could use keys and guitar," I told her.

"I've got just the guys for you."

I couldn't believe my luck, and thanked her profusely.

"What about a backup vocalist?" she asked. "I've got the perfect girl for the job."

"Bring her," I said, without a moment's hesitation.

A few days later, the whole group was exchanging animated greetings inside a small, dilapidated rehearsal studio.

"Are you all ready?" I asked, brimming over with excitement.

"Hell yeah!" came the reply, followed by a boisterous rendition of "Mama Needs a Girls' Night Out."

Since the songs on my album had been recorded one instrument at a time, it was the first time I'd heard a song of mine performed whole by a live band. I'd never felt anything like it in my life. It was akin to giving birth to a baby, without the physical pain. It was hard to keep tears of joy from spilling down my cheeks throughout the entire rehearsal.

A week later, it was time for us to pull off the impossible: play four of my songs at the Battle of the Bands, as if we'd been a band forever. With the help of my fashionable girlfriend Tiffanie, I'd put together a "star quality" outfit (a black-and-red beaded halter top with I-meant-to-do-that ratty jeans and high heels), and my long hair was blown out to shiny perfection. I felt like a million bucks.

The line to get into the club wound around the block, and the place was packed. A buzz filled the air. Brad was there, of course, along with the Bunco Girls, who held up signs that read Go Laura! and We Love You, Laura! How could we lose?

My band was slated to play first, the least desirable time slot. But no matter; we were jacked up and ready to rock, and so was the crowd. I came onstage and, once again, was plagued with shaking hands. But the moment I started to sing and the crowd began screaming, I forgot my nerves and just enjoyed the ride. And you know what? We killed it, though my adrenaline-fueled dancing was a bit over the top.

When our short set was over, we watched the other three acts. One of the bands, a group of guys about my age, was particularly good; they'd obviously played together a helluva lot. If we didn't win, I was pretty sure they would. Another guy was clearly a talented singer-songwriter, but the songs he'd selected to play were pretty low-key for an event like this, so I didn't think he was in contention.

The last band was led by a young, extremely handsome guy with a heartfelt voice. His sidekick guitarist, a guy in leather pants, no shirt, and an open vest, thrashed his long black hair around and thrust his pelvis gratuitously through every song, obviously trying to look like Slash but looking like Rico Suave instead. In contrast with the band's organic, boy-next-door front man, Rico Suave's inauthentic shtick was totally out of place and comical.

After the fourth and final band had played, the judges went into another room to deliberate, leaving the contestants to stand around, wringing their hands and clutching their stomachs.

Finally, the head judge called all four bands up to the stage to announce the winner, Miss America pageant–style: "Third runner-up is . . . " that low-key singer-songwriter guy. "Second runner-up is . . . " the band of thirtysomethings I had thought would win. Was that a good or bad sign?

It was down to my band and the good-looking young guy with the Rico Suave guitarist. "First runner-up is . . . Laura Roppé."

Damn. We were the runner-up—also known as the losers. (As Will Ferrell's Ricky Bobby says in *Talladega Nights,* "if you're not first, you're last.") That handsome young guy—with Rico Suave on guitar!—had won. We were crushed. We just couldn't understand it.

A little while later, as my bandmates and I signed pointless forms in the back office, promising to perform at Kenny Chesney's concert if the winner had to drop out, the head judge pulled me aside to let me know we'd put on a great performance.

"You were definitely the fan favorite," he conceded. "But that young guy is just a bit more . . . what the judges are looking for."

I was pretty sure that was code for "you're just too damned old."

I was disappointed—that was the truth. But pretty quickly, I was able to look on the bright side: Every band member had said to me that night, "I believe in your music, Laura. I'm on board." I might have lost the contest, but—*snap!*—I had just gained the Laura Roppé Band.

Chapter 31

My Dearest Jane,

I have been having dreams in which my children are in
peril and I must save them, or where people die senselessly.
I am doing so well to deflect my fears about mortality in my
waking hours. I would appreciate it if my subconscious would
please follow my conscious's lead.

Shortly after my second chemo infusion, it

was time for the annual Bunco Girls' Christmas party. I had not committed in advance. "I'll come if I feel up to it," I had promised. But, of
course, I wanted to go. I missed my life. I missed my Bunco Girls.

As luck would have it, on the day of the party, I felt like three
hundred bucks. I cooked up a big vat of mashed potatoes (my specialty) and hitched a ride to the party, about a mile away, with my
neighbor Tiffanie. This year, the party was hosted by much beloved

Bunco Girl Rebecca (who also happens to be the wife of my running partner, Mike). Her home was warm and inviting and decked with wreaths and candles, like a scene out of *It's a Wonderful Life.*

As I entered Rebecca's kitchen, the other Bunco Girls were already drinking wine and swapping animated stories. When they saw me, they "woohoo-ed" with joy and surrounded me in a group embrace.

I sat down on a kitchen stool, and normal party conversations resumed: "Christmas presents . . . holiday plans . . . kids . . . baking cookies . . . too much to do . . . " I tried to track the conversations, but I felt myself shutting down. My scalp was suddenly killing me, and I was beginning to feel nauseated.

We sat down for dinner. Happy conversation continued all around me. I ate my dinner quietly, crawling deeper and deeper into a dark hole, further and further away. Silverware was clinking on china. Laughter. Joking. Compliments about the food. I couldn't think of anything to add to the conversations around me. Hair loss? Fatigue? Fear of death? Buzzkills, all of them. Staying positive? I was tired of talking about that. Wrapping presents and Christmas shopping? I didn't care, to be perfectly honest. There was nothing to say. And then my hands felt clammy. The walls began closing in.

I slipped into the other room to pull myself back together. I could still hear the happy chatter from the dining room. I was all alone. I started to cry. And cry.

Brad.

After fumbling to retrieve my cell phone from my purse, I called Brad at home.

"Baby, come get me," I whispered. I didn't want the other ladies to hear me.

Brad didn't ask a single question. "I'm coming," he answered, and then he hung up the phone.

Two minutes later, Brad blasted into the room like Mr. Incredible, found me weeping in the living room, and whisked me out the front door. Though I was able to squeak out "I love you" and "I'm sorry" to my stunned friends between sobs as I left the house, I couldn't offer any explanation about what was happening to me. And, really, I didn't fully understand it myself.

But I did know one thing for sure: Brad, once again, was my hero.

A quiet Christmas with family came and went.

What a difference a year makes, I thought, recalling Sharon's Christmas party exactly one year before, when Matthew had first offered to demo the songs in my head. *Was that really only a year ago?*

On New Year's Eve 2008, Brad and I sat through my third chemo. *Happy New Year.* As I sat in my Barcalounger, a tube pumping poison into my arm, I made a list of my New Year's resolutions:

> *I resolve to do my best at this life, including following my passions, keeping my body healthy, and giving and receiving love with simplicity and honesty.*

> *I resolve to "say what I mean and mean what I say."*

I resolve to express my gratitude to all the people getting me through my treatments with love, meals, flowers, playdates for the girls, gifts, and emails.

And, finally, I resolve to beat cancer and never, ever hear those words "I've got bad news . . ." from a doctor ever again.

That night I was in bed, deathly sick, with faithful Buster at my side. At nine o'clock, Brad and the girls came in, flutes of apple cider in hand, to wish me Happy New Year, East Coast time, since the girls couldn't make it to midnight. At midnight, Brad came in again and whispered, "Happy New Year, my love" in my ear. But as I waged my fierce internal battle, I could barely register the tender moment.

Just as Dr. Hampshire had warned, each chemo infusion had become harder and harder as the toxins had accumulated. My body had begun to deteriorate. My red-blood-cell counts were becoming dangerously low. The fatigue was becoming unmanageable. I could not tolerate the shooting pains in my bones. I started relying on powerful pain medication to get me through the worst days. The meds helped, but they made me cloudy and listless. My appetite was nonexistent, and my taste buds didn't work right. Everything tasted weird and metallic. I lost weight. My eyes were sunken, and my skin had become gray. I had long since lost all the hair on my head and everywhere on my body, but now my eyelashes and eyebrows were starting to fall out, too. When I looked in the mirror, I did not recognize myself.

"How did I get here?" I asked my reflection aloud. It gave me comfort to hear my voice. I still *sounded* like me.

Many days as I lay in bed, I could hear the girls, coming in from school, downstairs with the baby sitter. I could hear them flinging their backpacks onto the floor, and the refrigerator door opening and closing. But I could not move. And then, the next thing I knew, there were warm hands on my cold, bald head. Caressing it. And then luscious, soft lips pressed against my hairless skin.

"Hi, Mommy," would come the little voice. "I love you."

"Crawl in, baby," I would say quietly, lifting up the corner of my bedspread. And whichever girl it was, sometimes both, would scootch right into bed with Buster and me, making my shivering, cold body feel warm again. I would touch their cheeks and inhale the smell of them, and I would thank God that six months earlier, I'd felt an inexplicable urgency to record an album. Thanks to that album, no matter what the future might hold, my voice would always be there to guide my little daughters in song:

Take my hand, little daughter, I'll tell you what I know
Won't be around forever, but I hope to see you grow
Into a beautiful woman with a child of your own
Hear my words, little daughter, you'll never be alone
Learn to play piano so your voice can soar and shine
Let the world hear your songs, and when I'm gone,
    please sing mine
Run into your fears, never run away
Don't waste a precious minute, learn right now to seize the day
Pain will come, as sure as you live and breathe
The hurt may rip your heart out and knock you to your knees

But be your mother's daughter, and know the sun will
  surely shine
Don't let the dark times steal your soul, tomorrow will be fine
If you're worried a man won't "let you,"
  then he's not the one for you
Find a man like Daddy who wants you to be you
You can talk about your dreams till kingdom come
But what you do, little daughter,
  that's where character comes from
Oh, I love you so, the greatest joy in my whole life
  is watching you grow

"Mommy, why'd this have to happen to you and not someone else?" Sophie asked one night as we pressed our bodies together in my bed.

"Honey, it might as well be me. If it were someone else, then that's someone else's mommy, and that wouldn't be any better, would it?" I answered. I had long since accepted that this was my mountain to climb.

Sophie considered this idea with the utmost seriousness. Her body went limp against mine. "You're right, Mommy," she finally declared, sounding weary. "I wouldn't want this to happen to anyone else's mommy."

Oh, Sophie. My eyes welled with tears.

Chapter 32

With all the recording on my album wrapped up, it was time for me to impersonate a supermodel for my album cover. My chosen photographer was Bil Zelman, a renowned photographer who'd shot countless album covers for Virgin Records. He met me at a remote mountaintop location outside San Diego, looking every bit like the rock 'n' roll photographer I'd envisioned.

I had brought several outfits to choose from, and I laid them out for Bil to peruse.

"I like that one," he said, pointing emphatically to a black, leg-revealing minidress covered in splashy sequins. "It's perfect."

I'd always been self-conscious about my skinny legs. Back in fifth grade, right after I'd transferred to a private school twenty miles from my neighborhood, I'd spent every afternoon riding my bike around a nearby park, hoping to befriend the kids from the local schools. One afternoon as I circled the perimeter of the park, trolling for friends and enjoying the sunshine in my snazzy tank top and Dolphin shorts, a group of boys playing flag football detected my loneliness like sharks smelling blood.

"Hey, Pencils! Hey, Olive Oyl!" they shouted to me. "How do you even ride a bike with legs like that? Your legs are gonna break!" They cackled with laughter.

I had no witty comeback.

I had always known my legs were on the skinny side, of course. But in that instant, in a sudden epiphany, I realized they were *freakishly* skinny. The full extent of their embarrassing ugliness dawned on me all at once. Speechless, I changed course on my bike and rode back home as fast as my stick legs could pedal.

For several years after that, I did not wear shorts, no matter what the weather. And that's saying a lot when you live in Southern California. When I finally succumbed to the sunshine and wore shorts again, I was pretty sure everyone was snickering at me behind my back. By then, though, I had simply resolved to suck it up.

And now this charismatic rock photographer was suggesting that I wear a leg-baring minidress—a dress that would display my chopstick legs in their full glory—for a photo that could become one of the defining pictures of my life.

"Hey, that one was my first choice, too," I responded without hesitation. It was like giving a high-five to my ten-year-old self.

Of course, since we were in the middle of the dusty countryside on a mountaintop, the aforementioned sequined ensemble seemed a completely inappropriate wardrobe choice. *Perfection!*

"Here, hold this," Bil said, handing me a purple wildflower he had just picked from the side of the road. "Now, just give me a second while I check the lighting."

"Sure thing."

I stood there holding that purple flower, waiting for Bil to begin shooting, passing the time by admiring how his curly hair gleamed in the spring sunshine. But, unbeknownst to me, Bil had been shooting the whole time I'd been standing there. After a moment, he looked at the small screen on his digital camera and smiled broadly.

"Hey, Laura, look at this," he called to me.

I hobbled over to Bil—quite a feat in six-inch heels on a bumpy dirt road—and squinted at the image on his camera screen. When my eyes settled on the picture before me, I smiled, too. There was my album cover.

When I finally got the big box of CDs back from mass duplication in August 2008, I ripped it open. And there I was, in my black minidress and towering heels, staring back at me. I touched the smooth, glossy CD cover in my hands and felt like weeping for joy.

A few days later, with a bit of luck, I managed to get my CD into the hands of "Little Tommy" Sablan, the producer of the highest-rated morning radio show in San Diego, and he shocked me by promising to listen to it.

The very next morning, the telephone rang. It was Little Tommy calling. "Turn on your radio," he said abruptly. "We're about to play 'Float Away.' The guys [the stars of the show, Jeff and Jer] are going to hear it for the first time on the air. They might love it, and they might hate it. Whatever the reaction, it'll be real. Good luck." And then he was gone.

I was shaking.

Brad, the girls, and I crowded around the radio, tittering with excitement. After a few lascivious (but not unappreciated) comments about my booby-leggy, purple-flower photo and some lampooning about the lengthy dedication to my family and friends on the album's inside cover (they were particularly amused by my mention of Grandpa Wayne-o), Jeff and Jer finally played "Float Away"—a song written by little ol' me—on the radio!

"She says I think I'll go home, turn off the telephone . . . " I heard myself sing through our stereo speaker. A tree had fallen in the forest, and tens of thousands of people were around to hear it.

When the song finished playing, Jeff and Jer's comedic tone had vanished. They said things like, "Wow!" and, "Where did this girl come from?" And then, best of all, they exclaimed, sounding genuinely surprised, "Our phones are lighting up!" Indeed, listeners were calling the station in droves to gush about the song. My song!

The first caller was a woman who could hardly speak through her sobs. "That song just spoke to me!" she cried.

"It told *my* story," another woman blubbered into the phone.

And the calls just kept coming and coming. Every single caller praised the song and said it had resonated with them. The avalanche of listener response to "Float Away" was overwhelming.

"Laura, can you come perform 'Float Away' for our listeners at our big listener party in a few weeks?" Jerry asked.

"Oh my God, yes!" was my immediate reply.

In late August 2008, I walked onstage at Jeff and Jer's listener party in front of 3,500 people—which felt like three million people to me—and performed "Float Away" with my band. My hands were shaking (again) as I held the microphone, but I sang from the bottom of my heart. And, in one of the most surreal moments of my life, I realized the crowd was singing my own song back to me. Thousands of people knew my song! I'd never felt a rush quite like it before.

"Hi Laura," an email from a "fan" in the UK began.

"I love your music. Do you ever plan to come to the UK to do any shows? Regards, John."

Isn't that sweet, I thought. And, in typical Laura fashion, I didn't hold my cards close to my vest when I replied:

> *Hi John, thank you for your nice email. I would love to come to the UK one day, but the truth is, I don't have the faintest idea how to make that happen! I released my album on my own, without a record label, and I don't have any connections within the music industry. If you know any-one who has connections in the UK music industry, I'd be grateful for any leads.*

Of course, I didn't know then that John, my UK fan, was actually the head of a record label based in London; he'd concealed his voca-tion until he'd gotten a sense of my personality. Luckily, he told me later, he'd been instantly charmed by my utter lack of pretense.

"Did you discover me through Jeff and Jer?" I asked, once I'd learned of John's true profession.

"No," John answered. "I found you myself, on the Internet."

Thank you, Internet.

Over the next several weeks, Brad and I negotiated the terms of a contract with John for the release and distribution of my album in the UK and Europe. John loved my entire album, he said, but "Float Away" in particular. The very first order of business would be for me to travel to the UK, probably in late October 2008, to shoot a music video for "Float Away" and to embark on a promotional tour throughout the country. *A music video?! A tour?!* My head was spinning.

"Brad," I asked breathlessly when I got off the latest phone call with John. "Can I go to the UK? Can you handle the girls while I'm gone? Can I go? Can I?"

Brad, the love of my life, the man who had loved me since I was fourteen years old, the man who understood me better than I understood myself, answered, "Absolutely." And then, in his best Cuban accent, he added, "Oh, Lucy, you're gonna get into the Copacabana, aren't you?"

Chapter 33

During those giddy weeks when Brad and I were negotiating my record deal with John from London, I felt it: a tiny, hard lump on the side of my left breast. I was confused. Had that been there all along?

I went to Brad, who was already in bed.

"Babe," I crawled into bed next to him. "Do you feel this?" I put his finger directly on the bump. "Has that always been there?"

Brad's face was pensive as he touched the spot where I had placed his finger. And then his face turned dark. "You need to go to the doctor about this right away," he ordered. "Tomorrow."

I'd had a clean mammogram right before getting my boob job two years earlier. "I think that's a bit of an overreaction, honey," I said. I wasn't the least bit worried, though I couldn't remember having felt that lump before. "I'm sure it's nothing."

But Brad insisted. "Promise me you'll go to the doctor about this tomorrow."

My calendar was loaded with lots of client meetings and court appearances the next day. I hesitated.

"Buddy, promise me," Brad repeated. "Tomorrow."

"Okay, okay. I promise." I knew that resisting Brad would be useless.

I called my doctor the next morning, if only to avoid Brad's persistent nagging on the subject, and was surprised she could fit me in right away.

"Well, there's definitely a lump there," Dr. Paula Dozzi confirmed as she examined my breast. "Do you have a history of breast cancer in your family?"

"No."

"Did you breastfeed?"

"Yes, both my girls."

"Do you exercise regularly?"

"Yes. I run." *A lot.*

"How is your stress level?"

"High." *But what else is new?*

"Well," Dr. Dozzi began, "based on your history and age, it's very unlikely that this is cancer. But there's definitely a pea-size lump there."

I nodded. Many of my girlfriends had discovered lumps in their breasts that had turned out to be calcifications or benign cysts. I was too young to get breast cancer, and I felt completely fine. And, truth be told, bad things didn't happen to me. I was sure it was nothing.

"Just to be on the safe side, though, I really want you to get a mammogram and also see a surgeon," the doctor continued. She wrote me a referral for the mammogram and gave me the surgeon's contact information. "I don't want to worry you, but I just want to be sure."

"Thanks," I said casually, stuffing the referral into my purse. "I'm not worried." I smiled to reassure her.

As directed, I made an immediate appointment for a mammogram—not because I was anxious about the lump, but because I am a Dudley Do-Right to my very core: I change the oil in my car at the designated mileage; I do homework exactly as assigned; I cross streets at crosswalks; I shake my head no when offered a joint at a party; and, of course, I always, *always* follow doctors' orders.

At the mammogram a week later, the technician pulled and squashed my saline-filled breasts into potato pancakes to get the images she needed.

"Please don't pop me," I implored her.

She laughed, mistakenly assuming I was joking. "Don't worry. I do this all the time."

When the mammogram results came back, the findings were "normal." There was indeed a round mass in my left breast (I didn't need a fancy machine to tell me that); however, so said the mammogram, the mass wasn't reading as cancerous.

I knew it! Brad had overreacted.

He wasn't convinced, though. Despite the mammogram results, he still wanted me to see the surgeon as soon as possible, as Dr. Dozzi had suggested.

Yes, I agreed, of course. But I wasn't in any rush. Work was unbelievably hectic at that time, as I tried to fend off a perfect storm of lawsuits against my loud-mouthed client, Frank, so I vowed to make an appointment as soon as I could find a convenient time. I really would.

That night, Dr. Dozzi called me at home.

"Laura," she said. "I got the mammogram results. That's good. But I wanted to remind you to please make an appointment with the surgeon right away. I want to get a surgeon's opinion on that lump."

I promised her I would see the surgeon. "And I'm not worried," I added truthfully.

But Brad *was* worried. Really worried. A week later, he went with me to the surgeon's office.

The surgeon examined my breasts and the mammogram results, and then went through the same list of questions Dr. Dozzi had asked.

"It's highly unlikely that this is cancer, based on all the information I have," he concluded. "But even if the chances of this being cancer are two percent, that's just too high to ignore. What I recommend are removal and biopsy of the lump. It's always better to be safe than sorry in these matters."

All I really heard him say was "two percent chance of cancer." In my mind, that was akin to "zero percent chance of cancer." But, of course, I did not disagree with his recommendation for lump removal and biopsy. I added only one caveat: "Just don't pop my boob when you're poking around in there with a scalpel, Doc." I smiled.

"I haven't popped one yet," he assured, but he didn't smile back.

I wasn't worried at all.

And then, fast-forward three weeks, and—*snap!*—I was falling down an endless well of so-sorry-to-inform-you phone calls from doctors, MRIs, blood tests, and hospital gowns—drowning in a torrent of tears as Brad and I learned that yes, I had breast cancer; and yes, it was triple negative; and yes, it was multiplying rapidly; and yes, it had spread outside my breast; and yes, I'd need surgery, chemotherapy, and radiation.

In the blink of an eye, I wasn't an undercover rock star anymore. I was a cancer patient.

In a sudden jolt of reality, I realized I had to call John from the record label to give him the news. Right? I had to do that . . . didn't I? Yes, I did. The honorable thing to do was let him out of the contract—a contract we had signed only days before that world-upending phone call from the surgeon.

Due to the eight-hour time difference between San Diego and London, I had to wait until early the next morning to call. I barely slept that night, anticipating having to make that call. All night, I felt like Anne Boleyn trapped in the Tower of London the night before her gruesome execution.

When I called John's office the next morning, a receptionist with a Bond Girl voice cheerfully patched me through with a fervent "good day!" When John came on the line, I awkwardly cut off the polite pleasantries.

"John," I said evenly, "I have some bad news. I just found out I have breast cancer." My voice was calm, but my heart was breaking inside. "I don't know what's going to happen to me." I took a deep breath. "John, I release you from the contract. You signed a girl with hair and boobs, and I might not have either of those much longer."

John did not hesitate. "Laura," he said in his clipped British accent, "I don't want to be released from the contract. And *I* certainly don't release *you*. Do whatever you need to do to get better. Take care of yourself. And when you're all better, and I know you will be, we'll have you over here to film that music video after all. Just do what you need to do to get better."

I cried tears of joy and relief all at once, which I much preferred to my recent torrent of anxious tears.

"Thank you, John. You're a saint," I whimpered, my voice breaking.

"Not really," he quipped. "I just really love your music."

Chapter 34

At age eight, one year after my parents had divorced, I sat on the bottom stair at my dad's new house, crying a river of tears, after having discovered that my Rubik's Cube had been relieved of one of its essential red blocks, courtesy of one of my brand-new stepsisters.

"What's wrong?" Dad asked, settling himself next to me.

Wordlessly, I held out the broken Rubik's Cube in my hand, a fresh round of sobs rising up from my raw throat.

"Laura," Dad said in a firm but gentle voice, "never cry over *things*. Cry over *people*. Things can be replaced."

Sage advice. I've never forgotten it. Indeed, I've repeated it to my own children many times as they've mourned headless Barbies and eyeless teddy bears.

But what do you do when someone *is* crying over a person? What do you say when the man you love with all your heart is sobbing uncontrollably at the thought of losing his wife, the love of his life? And, in particular, what do you say when that wife, that love of his life, happens to be you?

On the eve of my third chemo session, as Brad and I lay in bed, clutching each other even in our sleep, I was awakened by the sound of his crying.

I was half asleep. "Don't cry," I said quietly, fumbling in the dark to pat his arm. "It'll be all right."

But Brad did not respond.

I sat up in bed and touched his chest. I looked at his face. *Oh, my baby.* Brad was asleep. He was crying in his sleep. I exhaled sharply, overcome by a pang in my chest.

"Don't cry, baby," I whispered, smoothing his hair.

He didn't respond.

I rolled over to go back to sleep.

I closed my eyes. I opened them again. I sat up. A song was rushing into my head at full speed. I leaped out of bed and rushed to my desk.

Twenty minutes later, I shook Brad's shoulder. "Baby! Brad! Wake up!"

Brad opened his eyes, startled. An instant panic seized him. "What is it? What's wrong? Are you okay?"

"I'm fine, Birdy, I'm fine. You were crying in your sleep, baby."

Brad's expression said, *And so you woke me up?*

"A song just came to me!" I exclaimed, by way of explanation.

He looked groggy.

"Listen to this," I said. And in the darkness, I sang to him:

Don't cry, it'll be all right
I'll be your woobie
Hold on to me tight
Don't fret, I'm not leaving yet
I'm holding my ground
Won't let this thing get us, I promise
Baby, baby, you're my woobie, baby, baby, I'm yours, too
I don't want no other woobie, baby, all I want is you
I'm here, I'm not going anywhere
Even though I'm scared, I'm not feeling any fear
With you standing by my side
The monster can't hide
Gonna slap it upside the head
Baby, baby, you're my woobie, baby, baby, I'm yours, too
I don't want no other woobie, baby, all I want is you

"Buddy, I love it," Brad said, pulling me close to him. And then, completely contrary to my purpose in writing the song in the first place, he began to cry.

Chapter 35

Brad never even considered missing a single chemo infusion or doctor's appointment, even though countless friends and family offered to take his place.

"I want to be the one to hold your hand," he said firmly. "I'd *do* the chemo for you if I could."

Obviously Brad couldn't do that, and even if he could have, I wouldn't have let him. But there *was* something he could do for me, something I was too embarrassed to ask anyone else to do, something I'd never done in my whole life: hold the hash pipe for me when I finally inhaled my first hit of Mary Jane. Now, that's what I call being a caregiver.

A fellow cancer patient had given me a baggie full of marijuana as a gift. "It's the only thing that helps me," he had told me in a weary voice, totally unsolicited. "Maybe it'll help you, too."

Of course, given my lifelong abstention from drugs, and my

goody-two-shoes nature in general, I had been about to say, "No, thanks" to my benefactor. But then, for some reason, I had instead replied, "Thanks a lot."

Nonetheless, that little bag had remained securely hidden in my medicine cabinet for several weeks, until one night, after a particularly difficult chemo session, I crept downstairs once the girls were sleeping soundly in their beds and found Brad watching TV on the couch.

"Brad, will you help me?" I asked, holding up the baggie and the pipe.

Brad glanced up, and an amused grin washed over his face. "My pleasure."

If my new friend (i.e., my new drug dealer) had given me a rolled joint, I'd have known exactly what I was supposed to do: light it, stick it in my mouth, and inhale (unlike Bill Clinton). Simple. But I'd never seen this particular type of pipe thingamajiggy and bag of green buds before, and I needed a tutorial.

Now, don't get me wrong—I'd seen pot before. Way back when I was nine years old, I sat on the couch with Dad's new wife, Laila, as she watched *Fantasy Island*, all the while toking away on a big fat water bong. The hypnotic gurgle of the bong, and Tattoo shouting, "Da plane, da plane!" filled the smoky family room.

After a long inhale, Laila turned slowly to me, a vacant look in her eyes, and said, without a hint of irony or intentional humor, "You know who Mr. Roarke is, don't you?"

I shook my head. *Ricardo something*, I thought.

"He's God," Laila answered. And then she took a long, gurgling hit off the bong.

Not too long after that, Dad sat me down to tell me that he and Laila were kaput. "Some people have little capsules inside their heads, sort of like Tylenol capsules," he said. "And sometimes one of these capsules opens up and tiny beads spill out."

I looked at Dad quizzically, trying to make heads or tails of what he was trying to tell me.

"The problem is," Dad explained further, "sometimes the beads are . . . crazy beads. And that's what's going on inside Laila's brain," he summed up.

I understood pretty well: Laila's crazy beads had gotten loose and were rolling around inside her head.

And so my own fleeting, real-life Cheech and Chong movie came to an end.

But the damage had been done: I became an antidrug zealot, certain that one little puff of pot would decimate two million brain cells at a time and reduce me to a Mr. Roarke–worshipping ninny. And thus I primly declined each and every joint that was proffered to me throughout my teens and twenties, never entering my own personal Age of Aquarius.

After college, after I'd embarked on a career as a professional tight-ass, lighting up a doobie never occurred to me. And, of course, once I had become a minivan-driving mother of two, becoming dazed and confused was out of the question.

And that was why now, at age thirty-eight, I needed Brad's help to become a pothead. Really, this pipe and loose bag of buds didn't look anything like the water bong I'd seen in my childhood, and they didn't come with an instruction manual. Although Brad's last puff on a joint had been as a teenager almost two decades before, at least he'd had more experience with the stuff than I had.

Brad looked strangely elated. His straitlaced wife was finally going to join the rank and file and get stoned! No matter that I was bald and sickly; this was his chance to finally knock me off my holier-than-thou pedestal.

We went outside onto our patio into the chilly night air, where, after sitting me down at a table and wrapping me meticulously in a warm blanket, Brad gave me proper instructions.

"I'm going to put the buds into the pipe, and when I light it, you need to inhale deeply into your lungs. Okay?" I nodded, my eyes wide. "The hardest part for first-timers," he continued, "is inhaling deeply enough that the pot gets into their system. You can't just inhale into your mouth and throat; that'll just make you cough, and you won't feel anything."

"I can do it," I assured him. "Hit me."

Brad laughed. "Hit me," he echoed, and grinned.

He carefully packed the little mosslike balls of pot—or, as I like to say, weed, herb, Mary Jane, spliff, ganja, reefer, bud, dope, doobie, purple haze, devil's lettuce, hashish—into the pipe, and then he lit it with a match. *Ooh, that smell.*

Brad gently held the pipe up to my lips, and I inhaled. Deeply. And then I held the smoke in my lungs for what seemed a very long time.

The seal had been broken.

"Oh my God," Brad whispered. "You're a natural."

I laughed, and a white puff of smoke shot out of my mouth. And then I coughed. "I guess I've got big ol' singer's lungs," I reasoned. Or maybe I'd picked up a thing or two from watching my blink-and-you'll-miss-her stepmom, Laila.

My throat felt hot and scratchy, and my lungs hurt. I felt as if I'd just escaped from a burning building. *How the hell is this so alluring to everyone?* I wondered. But, hell, I had nothing to lose.

"Hit me again," I ordered.

Now that I'd given up my reefer V-card, I figured I might as well find out what all the fuss was about. And given the sickness and pain I was already feeling, killing two million brain cells didn't seem like such a travesty. I'd have sacrificed all of them to make the pain go away.

"This is hysterical," Brad whispered, as he held the pipe up to my lips again, and then we both started laughing uncontrollably, although we were careful not to make so much noise as to attract notice from our neighbors, a mere ten feet away, on the other side of the fence.

Perhaps you are wondering if Brad took the opportunity to smoke with me. He did not. You might not believe me, but it's true. Pot held no attraction for him, he said. And even if it had, he had two little girls sleeping upstairs who needed a sober parent in the house, as well as a cancer-stricken wife who'd just taken her first hit of weed at the age of thirty-eight. Who knew how I'd react?

Brad and I settled onto the couch to watch TV together before I inevitably drifted off to sleep. I was staring intently at the television, watching the medical drama *House*, when I heard Brad's garbled voice next to me, sounding as if he were standing in a distant wind tunnel.

"That was so funny," Brad mused about something that had just happened in the show.

I turned my dull gaze to him. "What was so funny?" I asked slowly, though I'd been staring at the television the whole time.

"Oh, honey, you are so stoned," Brad observed. And he was right.

But even in that state, I still felt absolutely horrible. Now, I was just feeling horrible *and* stoned, and my throat and lungs felt as if I'd just spent the night in a Las Vegas casino. For me, marijuana (even this strong stuff) was no match for the powerful chemo drugs coursing through my body. As it turned out, I much preferred the anti-nausea medications, painkillers, and sleep aids Dr. Hampshire gave me to combat the chemo's effects; at least with those, I didn't feel like my lungs were on fire. But, oh well, it was worth a shot. And, I must confess, it was a relief to hang up my long-standing goody-two-shoes for good.

Chapter 36

She says, this life's too heavy, I've reached the breaking point

If I check out now I can leave it all behind

And float, float away

But she hears the voice of her little girl

Only thing that matters in this whole world

Gotta find a way not to fade away

Hold on, for one more day

She's not sure how she got to this place,

  the world is crashing down

Gotta have faith it'll be all right,

  too much to lose if she loses this fight

Baby growing up ashamed all her life if she goes away,

  if she fades away

Won't float away, no! Won't float away

Hold on, for one more day

Hold on, for one more day

When I wrote my song "Float Away," I

was six months shy of my cancer diagnosis. Cancer was still someone else's sad misfortune, something that would never happen to me. In fact, I had never faced a defining hardship in my own life, though, of course, I had experienced personal heartaches and disappointments. "Float Away" was what came out of me when I allowed myself to feel others' struggles vicariously.

Way back when Brad and I were teenagers, we were driving south toward Mexico, intent on reveling in a carefree day of surfing (Brad), sunbathing (me), and lobster, when we spotted a young woman clinging to the *outside* of a chain-link fence on a freeway overpass, just before the Mexican border.

The girl was perched on a three-inch-wide strip of cement, clutching the chain-link fence at her back and looking down at the rushing cars twenty feet below. There was no question in our minds what she was doing out there on that precarious ledge, her skirt billowing above the speeding traffic below.

"Pull up onto that overpass, right next to that girl," I ordered Brad, and he did, holding his breath in anticipation.

I had never been trained in crisis management, and I didn't know the recommended protocol in such a situation. But what I did know was this: *I was pissed.*

Wordlessly, I stomped out of the car, slamming the door behind me, and marched directly toward that shivering girl.

The roar of the passing traffic below us forced me to shout, even though we were standing mere feet apart. "Hey!" I called out in a stern voice. "You there!"

She turned to look at me with wide brown eyes.

Oh, she's younger than I'd thought. She was about my age.

"Get down from there and come over here this instant!" My tone was indignant. *"Right now!"*

But she didn't budge. She just stared at me for a few seconds and then turned her dull gaze back to the freeway.

I was miffed. *How dare she!*

"You know, you're not allowed to be there!"

Still no reaction.

I inched closer to the girl, until I was standing about a foot away from her, just behind her right shoulder, on the safe side of the chain-link fence. She didn't react to my advancement, but instead maintained her blank stare at the onrushing traffic.

"Do you speak English?" My tone was not gentle; it was bossy. Still no response. *"¡Ven acá este minuto! ¡Está prohibido!"* I shouted with authority, showing off my many years of Spanish-language studies.

Without acknowledging me, the girl with the big brown eyes tilted her gaze to her right, toward the end of the chain-link fence, twenty yards away, and then slowly began to inch her way across the length of the fence, back toward the safety of the overpass. She finally arrived at the open edge of the fence and stepped gingerly onto the sidewalk. For just a moment, she stood about a foot from me, both of us now on the safe side of the fence, and our eyes met.

How could you even think of doing such a horrible thing? And then I felt my heart soften. *Why do you feel so hopeless?*

Her big brown eyes flashed at me one last time, and then she ran away without a word.

I stood rooted to my spot on the sidewalk, as a loud semitruck rattled past me on the freeway below.

I climbed back into the car, where Brad had watched this drama unfold from the driver's seat.

"What did you say to her? That was crazy!" he exclaimed, but I was too stunned to respond.

He didn't push me for a response. Instead, he silently started the car and pulled back onto the road, shaking his head in disbelief. I looked out the car window, lost in my thoughts as our car merged into traffic again. She was nowhere to be seen.

I pulled down the visor mirror above my car seat and gazed at my own brown eyes. But all I could see were that girl's haunting brown eyes staring back at me.

It was then, and only then, that I thought to myself, *Holy crap*.

Throughout the twenty years after that day, I thought about the girl with the empty brown eyes many times. Had she returned to the bridge to complete her mission five minutes after we'd left? Or maybe the next day? There was no shortage of freeway overpasses in the world. Or had she gone straight home to swallow a bottle of pills?

I had somehow managed to shame her off that bridge that day, but I'd done nothing to give her hope, to change her heart. I had merely distracted her for a brief moment, like swatting at a fly buzzing around a picnic feast.

As time went by, I realized the girl on the overpass was not alone, that occasional strangers were drowning in despair and longing all around me. A passing glance from a stranger entering the bank jolted me with a sudden, but palpable, flash of sadness. At the park, when I witnessed a mother pushing her young child on a swing, I could *feel* her hopelessness as surely as if she'd whispered, "Help me" into my ear. As surely as if she'd been standing on a freeway overpass.

And each time a stranger's hopelessness whispered to me, the idea blossomed inside me just a little bit more: I wanted to give them hope. I wanted to make a lasting impact.

When "Float Away" started to make its way around the world through the magic of radio and the Internet, I began receiving emails and cards from people who had heard the song. One woman wrote to tell me she had just lost her young husband in a tragic boating accident. "I am struggling to carry on," she said, "for the sake of my three young boys." Someone had played "Float Away" in her young-widows support group, she wrote, telling the group, "You have to listen to this song." After that first day, she had listened to the song fifty times in a row, she wrote in her email, and it had helped her get through each day.

Another woman wrote to tell me that every day, she had stolen away from her family to drown her sorrows in a bottle of wine. "No one knows my secret," she wrote to me, "but your song is giving me the strength to seek treatment."

A man wrote that his girlfriend was battling cancer and he had been playing the song for her every day throughout her treatments. "Your song gives her strength to get through the worst days," he wrote. "Thank you."

Back when I received these beautiful notes, only a few months before my own life was torpedoed by the unthinkable, I was deeply moved, of course, but I was not one of those people. I read Brad every email and note, my voice cracking and catching with each word, but I stood safely on my side of the chain-link fence.

I can help others through my music, I thought. Surely this was my higher purpose. Why me, I didn't know, when I hadn't suffered a catastrophic setback in my own life, but it felt right, like the fulfillment of some lifelong potential.

It did not occur to me then that in the coming months, I would cling desperately to hope in my own life, too. No, I thought, I would be the purveyor of inspiration for others, through my music; but in my own life, I would hopscotch across the clouds as I'd always done. Because, you know, bad things never happened to me.

But, oh, how life can turn on a dime with just one phone call! One little phone call from that damned surgeon, and I had been ripped from the safety of the sidewalk and pushed onto a concrete ledge overlooking an overpass. I had become *one of them,* one of *those other types of people.* Pitiable. Pitiful.

And now, having reached my fourth chemo infusion, the half way mark in my arduous chemotherapy regimen, a milestone I'd thought would be cause for celebration and high-fiving, I felt nothing but despair. I wasn't fist-pumping the air at reaching the halfway mark. No, I was decrying the interminable second half yawning before me.

The glass was half empty.

At night, I had started to have recurring dreams in which my girls were in some form of peril—Chloe falling off a towering ledge, Sophie being swept out to sea. And in each dream, there I stood, mere inches away from my endangered child—powerless, ineffectual, reaching, reaching, screaming, crying. Impotent. Each morning when I awoke, my heart felt bruised from the previous night's battering.

The glimmering memory of my prior self, my vital and powerful self, was becoming faded and cracked. I was beginning to feel . . . hopeless.

After coming home from my fourth chemo infusion, the halfway point of a grueling marathon, a milestone I'd expected would elicit excitement and a sense of accomplishment, I stood in the shower, letting the hot water pound my scrawny back, and I cried deep, heaving sobs.

I could give up, I thought suddenly. *I have the power to make it all go away.*

This was a novel thought. I had the power to make the pain and dreariness go away!

This wasn't a movie. This was real life. And it sucked. Hard. And I wanted out.

It was my prerogative to end it all! All I had to do was stop fighting! Why had I been fighting so hard—not just now, against cancer, but all my life? I'd always been so fierce, so focused, so accomplished. Never a quitter! Never half-assed! And where had it gotten me? Here. To *this.* What was the point in any of it? Why keep fighting? What was the big whoop about survival, anyway? Easy come, easy go.

Just succumb already, Laura! All the pain will melt away!

An entire lifetime of pushing, and pressing, and proving—swinging my machete through dense jungles of my own making (à la Michael Douglas in *Romancing the Stone)*—and I suddenly recognized my own power: I could simply let go, and . . . fade away.

The path of least resistance. I'd never taken that path before. It sounded . . . relaxing. Like a steam bath.

What difference would it make, really? One less person on Planet Earth out of, what, billions? Just one less person . . .

I drew a frowny face in the steam on the shower door.

Poor me.

What was happening to me? This was so unlike me!

The hot shower water beat down on me, mixing with the tears streaming down my face.

"Hold on, for one more day . . . " I sang in the shower, my voice almost inaudible. "Hold on for one more day." I sang more loudly. "Hold on for one more day! Hold on for one more day!" It was a battle cry.

I waited. Wasn't this song—*my song*—supposed to summon the angels straight down from heaven? Wasn't this song—this beacon of light and hope—supposed to lift me out of my darkest moment? Wasn't this song supposed to *inspire* me?

I waited.

"Hold on for one more day," I said flatly, this time in a speaking voice.

Apparently not.

Chapter 37

My Dearest Jane,

*I cried yesterday and today. I was not crying about the big-
picture, "I don't want to die" stuff. I was crying just for the here
and now. I feel so ugly. For all my bravado, I am so very sick
of looking at my bald head. And I hate the smell. Do you smell
that, too? I feel like I smell my chemo all the time—on my skin,
on my clothes, on my sheets, in my stuffy room. I open the win-
dows, I change the sheets, but I still smell it. I am such a grab-
life-by-the-horns person, and all I do nowadays is lie there and
stink. I had put lots of stock in this halfway point. And instead
of feeling jubilant at arriving here, I feel overwhelmed that
I've still got four to go. Four! That seems very long indeed. You
know I am not usually like this, Jane. I'll be better tomorrow,
I promise. I know when I see my doctor tomorrow he'll have a
way of making me forget the self-pity.*

When Dr. Hampshire entered the examination room, he could plainly see I was on the verge of crying. It was unlike me. I was his upbeat, positive patient. His role model for other patients. A force of nature! A limitless well of strength. Not a beaten-down, can't-get-my-ass-up-again quitter.

"What's up?" he asked.

"It feels like such a long road," I whimpered, the wax paper crinkling beneath me on the examination table. "I can't see the end." My voice was breaking. "I'm starting to . . . " I couldn't bear to finish the sentence. *Give up.*

Dr. Hampshire looked me in the eye. He knew.

"Laura," he said firmly, "you are the strongest person I know. Do you hear me? You can do this."

"But . . . " I began, intending to let him in on my secret. I was not strong. I was a quitter. I was a big fat quitter!

"All you have to do is keep showing up, Laura, and I'll do the rest," Dr. Hampshire continued. He got up from his desk chair and stood beside the examination table. He touched my forearm. "Laura, the road is already shorter than it was yesterday. Every single day, you are one step closer to being finished. And when you are finished, you will be cured, and you will never look back. You will live a full life; you will raise your daughters." And then, with an intensity befitting the skilled down-from-the-ledge talker he was, Dr. Hampshire added, with absolute medical authority, "And—you—will—be—famous."

Against my will, I cracked a smile and chuckled, even as tears trickled down my cheeks.

One less person on Planet Earth out of billions? Bullshit. I would not go quietly into that good night. No, I would fight tooth and nail to make it to my 103rd birthday.

"Doc, there are just no guarantees," I responded, my spirit beginning to flicker back. "About fame, that is."

Dr. Hampshire laughed. "No, but some things are just inevitable."

Indeed, we both knew he could make no guarantees about any of it—life, death, health, fame. But it didn't matter. Dr. Hampshire had the audacity, the compassion, in a world full of lawsuits and insurance companies and limits of liability, to promise to cure me, his patient on the brink of hopelessness.

And just like that, by doing so, he took the machete from my limp and blistered hand, and he began swinging and hacking, clearing a pathway through the dense jungle, just for me.

Even before my winning bingo card came up with all the right letters—C-A-N-C-E-R!—I'd always been fearful of death. Well, actually, not *death* so much as *dying*. I wasn't afraid to be dead so much as I didn't want to experience a gruesome and painful death.

There were a million possibilities for my eventual death, and some were downright horrifying. A terrifying car crash? Or, worse, a plane crash, with plenty of time to anticipate the ultimate impact? A serial killer, maybe?

Or perhaps I'd win the lottery (as I was entitled to, after all) and pass in my sleep at the ripe age of 103. Yes, I concluded each time precancerous thoughts of mortality danced in my head like sugarplum fairies in *The Nutcracker*, yes, I would die a very old woman, in my sleep, while wearing a white cotton nightgown (with pretty little eyelets trimming the bottom hem), my long gray hair brushed beautifully across the crisp white pillowcase. And I wouldn't feel a thing. It would be just like sleeping.

But once Brad and I started having babies, the accepted standards of parental care and responsibility obligated us to at least consider the possibility that one or both of us would make an unexpected, early departure, and most likely in a manner not including a white cotton nightgown with pretty eyelet trim. And, worse yet, we had to *plan* for this morbid possibility.

And so, back when Chloe was an infant, Brad and I trudged off to the office of our estate planner to sign a thick stack of useless documents that we would never need in real life, just so we could pat ourselves on the back and boast smugly to our yuppie friends, "We've put everything into a living trust, just in case. Haven't you?"

"Sign here, here, and here," the estate planning attorney instructed me. "And Brad, you sign here, here, and here."

Brad and I looked at each other, amazed at how adult we'd both become. We were ready for every contingency now—even our premature deaths, however inconceivable that possibility seemed.

"If I go first, Brad," I blurted, overcome with anxiety about future catastrophes, however hypothetical, "I would want you to remarry and find love again."

I stared at him expectantly, basking in my Mother Teresa–ness, awaiting his equally loving reply.

Without missing a beat, though, he replied, "Not me. If I go first and you remarry, I will haunt you like a poltergeist."

I laughed—as I always did at Brad's zingers—but then I rolled my eyes for the estate planner's benefit.

Actually, Brad's possessiveness thrilled me. I reveled in the thought that even in the afterlife, he would be infinitely unable to relinquish me to another man.

And now, only a few years after signing those estate planning documents, on the night after Dr. Hampshire had promised to cure me (presumably against the advice of the hospital's legal department), Brad and I lay in bed together, holding hands. Since hearing Dr. Hampshire's confident words, I'd felt the weight of the world lifted off me. Quitting was no longer an option.

And yet, I realized, there was no going back to my precancer state of bliss. I'd never again assume I'd make it to 103. I'd never again assume I'd make it through next year, for that matter. Now, suddenly, unexpectedly, the odds that I might precede Brad in death weren't quite as long as they'd once been.

"If I die," I said quietly, holding Brad's hand in the moonlit room, "I'm gonna hang around you and the girls in the afterlife, watching you, protecting you, and continuing to love you." Brad didn't say anything, so I continued, "I'll send you signs I'm there with you. If you don't see the signs, I'll be frustrated and bang my head against the wall. Well . . . my *proverbial* head against the *celestial* wall. You know what I mean." Still nothing from Brad. "So please, Buddy," I pleaded, "be alert and acknowledge me so that I can be at peace." I blinked back tears. This had been very difficult for me to say, but it had to be done.

Brad turned to look at me in the moonlight, without speaking for a brief moment. "Babe," he finally said, "I don't listen to you when you're alive. What makes you think I'll listen to you when you're dead?"

Chapter 38

My Dearest Jane,

The other day, I was not feeling well but had to mail
something. When I entered the mail store, the clerk was already
helping someone else, but she said to the lady she was helping,
"Ma'am, do you mind if I just help this lady [me] and then get
back you?" The "ma'am" was about to protest but then turned to
look at me. She saw my gray complexion and my head scarf and
said, "Of course not." Then she smiled at me and gave me I-am-
sorry-for-you eyes. Being a cancer patient has its perks.

Although my long brown wig had sounded
like a great idea before I lost my hair, once I was as bald as a cue ball,
it turned out I preferred myself au naturel. I never wore that pretty
brown wig. Not even once.

When I went out, I wore a simple scarf on my head, which, I quickly learned, was akin to stamping CANCER PATIENT on my forehead. But hey, it was easier for me than pretending everything was hunky-dory.

Looking like a cancer patient had its perks. (Occasional line cuts, for example.) But it also had its drawbacks: I was never just "some lady" anymore—a lady buying stamps at the post office. A woman unloading her groceries from a cart. No, even while performing simple errands, I was "the lady who is fighting bravely for her life." I was Susan Sarandon in *Stepmom*, courageously preparing her children for their future with Julia Roberts. A swelling, symphonic soundtrack followed me all the time, everywhere I went.

I often elicited reactions from passersby when I was out and about. Sometimes they turned away. Maybe I was an uncomfortable symbol of mortality, or perhaps a reminder of a heroic battle a loved one had fought. At the other extreme, people sometimes stared at me meaningfully, as if to say, *Hang in there* or, occasionally, *I've been there.* My return gaze always said, *Don't worry about me. I'm a fighter.*

Maybe I was just imagining all of these telepathic conversations, but I could hear them just the same.

At Chloe's first T-ball practice one chilly afternoon, a fellow mother, whom I'd never met before, approached me. Without preamble or ramp-up, she sidled up to me and stage-whispered, "You must really cherish every moment with your kids now."

Her eyes were moist.

Oh, wow, she thinks I'm dying, I thought. *And soon.*

Well, no, I don't cherish every moment with my kids now, as a matter of fact. Sometimes, especially when they're whining, they still annoy the crap out of me.

"Yes," I said to my new, nameless best friend, this unexpected shoulder to cry on, matching her intensity with my own urgent stage whisper, "yes, I really do." And then, just for good measure, I sighed deeply and shot her a meaningful glance.

I wanted to leave. I didn't want to be a walking emblem of mortality that day. I just wanted to watch Chloe's haphazard attempts at swinging a much-too-heavy baseball bat.

But really, what did I expect? What was this woman supposed to do in my presence? Ignore me? Or make idle chitchat? Can a person talk lightheartedly—about *American Idol*, perhaps—with someone she presumes is dying? With someone who is dying, talking about anything other than matters of life and death—about cherishing one's children—would be downright petty, right?

Maybe so. But I just couldn't be lofty and intense every minute of every day. At least not at T-ball, anyway.

The thing was, despite my physical appearance, despite all the infusions and doctor's appointments and medicine and weird smells and metallic tastes in my mouth and pain and nausea, I still felt like plain old me on the inside. I may have looked like a wraith, a gray phantom floating through life in a head scarf, but I was still me. The problem was, in my cancer patient disguise, no one could discern the undercover rock star held captive inside me. She had ceased to exist to the outside world. All anyone could see was this . . . this stupid . . . *container.*

Well, everyone, that is, except that weird guy in the grocery store parking lot a few days before.

I had just come out of the grocery store, gray as granite, wearing my head scarf and Jackie O. sunglasses, when a man in the parking lot approached me.

"Hi," he greeted me.

"Hello," I replied politely, though the thought of chatting with a stranger in a parking lot made me want to set my hair on fire. (Just a little cancer humor for you.)

"Do you shop here a lot?" he asked.

I figured this was his well-meaning attempt to convey his best wishes to the (presumably) dying lady, but I'd reached my "well-meaning attempt" quota for that week, and I was tired.

"Yes," I responded. "I shop here all the time." *Please get to the part where you encourage me to stay positive. I need to go to bed.*

"I really like your scarf," he said then, zeroing in on the singular thing about me that was compliment-worthy. What else could he have said—"I really like your gray pallor; it reminds me of dolphins, and I just love dolphins"?

Then something in the way he looked at me, just for an instant, caused me to realize he was *flirting* with me. But that was impossible.

"Thank you," I replied to his compliment, increasingly wary.

"Yeah, I saw it from across the parking lot, and I just wanted to tell you that."

"Thanks," I said again. Was there a point to this conversation? I was just so damned tired. I started to walk away. "Have a great day."

"So, um," he continued, stopping me dead in my tracks—and by that I mean he caused me to *stop walking,* just to be clear (a little more cancer humor for you)—"can I get your phone number?" he continued. "Maybe we could go out sometime?"

Long, awkward pause. I looked at him as if he had feet for hands.

Finally, my voice came: "Wow, thank you. That's sweet. But, I'm . . ."—*bald underneath this headscarf, you dumbass*—"married."

And then I ripped off my head scarf, leaped at him like a mountain lion on a jogger, and shouted, "How ya like me now, sucka!"

No, I didn't. But I wanted to.

Could he *really* have no idea he was talking to a just-about-to-crumple-to-the-ground-without-an-ounce-of-energy-left-in-her-sad-sack-body cancer patient? If so, he was the stupidest man alive. Or, alternatively, had this gentleman *knowingly* hit on such a pitiful creature? If so, he was a saint . . . or a total perv.

Ogled, I reminded myself. *It's always better to be ogled than "ma'am-ed." And yet in this instance,* I thought in a flash, *I think I'd rather be "ma'am-ed."*

Of course, Brad and the girls ignored my container, too. Despite my shocking physical transformation over the past several months, they still, thankfully, saw just me. Wife. Mommy. Me.

Indeed, Brad continued to tease me as mercilessly as he had before cancer, displaying absolutely no regard for the inspirational, saintly creature I had become.

"Hey, Elmer Fudd," he said to me at the dinner table one night, "pass the butter."

"Hellooo," I responded, "you're not supposed to tease me, Buddy. I have *cancer,* you know." I made the universal "duh" gesture with both hands.

"Babe, if I stop teasing you, *then cancer will have won,*" he retorted.

And he was right.

Damn. I hated it when Brad was right.

I walked Buster along a dirt trail by my house. The poor dog was becoming a bit rotund after spending so much time lounging in bed with me. I let him off-leash, and he immediately darted ahead to chase a bunny (or perhaps a leaf), but then rocketed right back to my side with (what I imagined to be) a gleeful *woohoo!* He repeated this dance over and over again.

In the third round of this game, when Buster looked up at me with his *woohoo!* expression, it hit me: Buster didn't see my physical appearance. He just saw *me.* I got that electric-current feeling that comes to me on occasion. *My identity has nothing to do with my physicality,* I thought. *I am not my container.*

Indeed, my whole life, this lesson had followed me around, poking me on the shoulder, urging me to listen. Back when I was thirteen years old, after arriving home from my preppy private school and throwing my backpack onto the floor, I changed from my good-girl clothes into a black shirt and leggings, wrapped a metal-studded belt around my hips (tiny as they were at the time), and smeared black lipstick on my lips. And then, with great care, I teased and shellacked my thick hair straight up into a "fauxhawk."

I assessed myself in the mirror: I was the Misunderstood Outsider—the prototype for Ally Sheedy in *The Breakfast Club,* a year before that movie existed. And then, in this getup, at precisely three o'clock in the afternoon, I embarked on the fifteen-minute walk up the hill, past the nearby junior high school, purportedly for an ice cream cone at Thrifty.

At ten past three o'clock on the dot, as planned, I passed the junior high school, just as the end-of-day bell sounded. As a swarm of kids leaving campus passed by, two or three of them heckled me: "Loser! . . . Hey, ugly! Go home!"

I kept walking past, glaring in seemingly angry defiance of my detractors.

All I want is an ice cream cone! I am not an animal!

But my angry glare was as much performance art as my hair. Really, I was amused and fascinated, much like an animal behaviorist studying an animated clan of orangutans. It tickled me to know that this outsider girl with the outrageous hair and black lipstick, the girl mocked as a "loser" by the "cool" kids, was actually a straight-A student from a preppy private school.

The next day, I followed my Ally Sheedy walk of shame with a second trek, dressed in my usual "honor student" clothes. This time when I walked past the school at the sound of the bell, boys drunk on their own newly awakened testosterone greeted me with smiles and flirtatious hellos.

Dummies, I thought. *I'm the same girl who came through here yesterday looking like Elvira*. It was the first time I distinctly thought, *Don't judge a book by its cover*.

And now, over twenty years later, I stood naked in front of my bathroom mirror, staring at my chemo-ravaged body, and the disconnect between my insides and outsides had never been more jar-ring: In this condition, my outsides, my container, actually looked a helluva lot like a Playboy Bunny—at least from the neck down. Since I'd lost so much weight, my fake boobs, initially sized for a bigger frame, were now disproportionately large and my hips had vanished. And, to top off this centerfold illusion, I was hairless. Everywhere. It looked like I'd had the world's most immaculate Brazilian wax. The image was unmistakable: I was a centerfold.

But how could this be? I was battling cancer, for Pete's sake. This "perfect" body was pickled in poisons! And yet wasn't this the very look American women were starving themselves to achieve? Here I was, finally looking like Pamela Anderson for the first time in my life, achieved as a by-product of being infused with the most toxic chemi-cals known to modern medicine!

And then here was the kicker, the coup de grace, the giveaway that all was not as it seemed: When I looked at myself from the neck up, I was a bald Bride of Chucky, a sunken-eyed zombie in search of brains to eat. I'd never looked worse in my entire life.

I had to laugh.

Don't judge a book by its cover, Laura.

It was an indisputable, hit-me-over-the-head life lesson in how little the physical body reflects the inner soul.

I am not my container.

Chapter 39

I was a hamster on a Thursday wheel.
Every other Thursday was Chemo Time, and the "off" Thursdays in
between set off a countdown for the next Thursday's dreaded infusion.
Each week was blending into the next, and I was starting to forget
who I'd been before this nightmare had started.

But then, on the "off" Thursday following my sixth chemo, just
as I was emerging from yet another week from hell, Little Tommy
from the *Jeff & Jer* radio show—the popular San Diego show that had
first aired "Float Away" six months earlier—reached out his hand and
pulled me off the wheel.

"Do you feel well enough to come down to the studio tomorrow
to update our listeners about you?" he asked.

Does Dorothy wear ruby slippers?

As it turned out, I'd remained somewhat of a listener favorite
since that first avalanche of positive response, and Jeff and Jer had

continued to update their audience on the twists and turns of my life. A few months earlier, I'd told their listeners about my then-recent diagnosis and upcoming treatment in an on-air telephone interview. It had been October—Breast Cancer Awareness Month—so I'd described in detail how I'd discovered the lump on my own.

"The mammogram came back as normal," I had warned. "Make sure you ladies do your self-examination."

Upon learning of my illness back then, fans of the *Jeff & Jer* show had inundated me with emails of well wishes and prayers.

And so when Little Tommy called right after my sixth chemo infusion to invite me down to the studio, I didn't hesitate.

Brad drove me to Jeff and Jer's studio at Clear Channel Radio—a behemoth radio conglomerate that blasts radio shows to the masses all over the country.

"Babe, I'll be fine," I told him. "You don't have to drive me."

"Nah, I'm coming," Brad declared. "You might be too wiped out afterward to drive, and I want to be on the safe side." And, of course, I knew, he didn't want to miss this exciting experience.

I was thrilled he was coming.

When we arrived at the studio building, Little Tommy welcomed us with big hugs in the hallway outside the studio. After a moment, when the show had broken for a commercial, Tommy led me into the studio, leaving Brad to watch the excitement through the window in the producer's booth.

The show's stars greeted me warmly as I put my big black headphones on over my head scarf. After a quick commercial break, we were live on-air (or "in the air," as Jeff and Jer liked to say).

First things first: Jeff played "Float Away" and another song of mine, "Sing a Love Song"—it never got old hearing my songs on the radio!—and I chatted with the show's hosts about the upcoming release of my music in the UK.

"When I'm all done with my treatment, I'm gonna go to England to shoot a music video!" I gushed. I sounded like a wallflower who's just been asked to dance by the captain of the football team—definitely not "acting like ya been there before." But I didn't care if my euphoria was over the top—they had given me the gift of feeling like my old self again, and it was exhilarating.

When Jeff asked me how I was holding up through treatment, I assured everyone I was staying positive, and they were happy to hear it.

"You're an inspiration," they said.

I didn't feel like an inspiration, though. In fact, I felt unabashedly selfish, reveling in self-centered glee at the chance to feel like myself again. If only for a day.

A few days after the radio interview, I was standing in line at Costco to buy snacks for Chloe's T-ball team. When I handed my membership card to the cashier and she saw my name printed at the bottom, she jerked her head up and gasped, "You're *Laura Roppé?* I love your music! I listen to you on *Jeff & Jer* all the time!" And then she craned her head around me to peer down the line of waiting customers and yelled, "Do you all know who this *is!?* This is *Laura Roppé!*"

The cashier then came around to my side of the conveyor belt and gave me an enthusiastic hug.

"I'm a five-year breast cancer survivor," she whispered in my ear, squeezing me for extra emphasis. "You're gonna get through this. Hold on for one more day, honey. Hold on for one more day."

As tears of gratitude filled my eyes, I squeezed her right back.

Chapter 40

Dear Laura,

Mine and Adam's marriage is over. It's been coming awhile. Things weren't great before I found out I had cancer, but I was just coasting along, as you do, and thinking that it wasn't good but it was tolerable, and potentially better than the alternative—i.e., having to start over again on my own. However, what the cancer has done was to make me realise that life is just way too short and that I don't want to not be happy.
Love, Jane xx

My Dearest Jane,

Big news, girlfriend. But I am not surprised at how cancer gives a person clarity coupled with unparalleled ability to act on it. Just as you've had an epiphany about your feelings for Adam, I've had my own: I cannot live without Brad. I want to grow old with him. I can understand completely if cancer doesn't cause that reaction how starkly you must feel that. It has been thrilling for me to realize that the only changes I want to make through all this are: (1) pursue music in earnest, and (2) never, ever practice another day of law in my life. So, really, I've done the same thing you've done, just in another context. I am here for you, come what may. I am just wishing you a full and happy life.

XOXOXO Laura

Dear Laura,

I love that you get what's going on in my life. Up to now, you're the only one who does. Everyone else thinks the cancer has "caused" the decision. But it hasn't; it's just acted as an enabler to facilitate my choices. It's not because of the cancer that I have made the choice I have. It's because of the cancer that I can't not act on how I feel.

Jane xx

And the truth was, though I worried for

Jane and felt sorry for Adam's heartbreak, I did understand. It might have seemed shocking for a woman to leave her husband while in the midst of cancer treatments, but I understood that Jane's pretenses had melted away and she'd lost the ability to lie to herself. About anything. I felt the same way.

Of course, we'd never had a guarantee of a long life, but we'd previously had the *illusion* of a guarantee. We'd put money away in our retirement plans for when we turned sixty-five. We'd planned to take a dream vacation—one day—perhaps after the kids had left the house. But now, after having been touched by a potentially deadly disease, our illusions were shattered. No matter how upbeat we remained, no matter how many times we gave two thumbs up in response to someone's rally cry "Stay positive!"—in the dark recesses of our minds, we could hear the doctor say, "It's back." And with that possibility hanging over our heads, the pressing question was: *What do I want my life to look like if that day of reckoning comes?* I understood that Jane was creating the life she wanted, no matter what the cost.

In my own way, I, too, was making bold decisions about the remainder of my life, no matter how long or short that was.

"When this is over, I can't go back to practicing law," I told Brad defiantly. "If I do, I'll have cancer again within two years."

Brad looked bewildered. He saw that I wasn't being hypothetical. And whether my prediction was true or not, it was clear I genuinely believed it.

I had finally embraced a fundamental truth about myself, no matter what the cost: I'm all heart, baby.

Take that, head!

The girls and I lay in bed together, creating our List of Things To Do Together This Summer. We knew that by summertime I would be finished with treatment. I would have hair. And I would be able to spend each and every day with my girlies, unlike in years past, when I had always worked at least several days per workweek. It was uplifting to us all to picture us happily enjoying a summer day together.

"How about a picnic?" Chloe contributed to the list.

"What else?" I prodded.

"The beach," Chloe said.

"Sea World?" Sophie added.

"That sounds fun!" I exclaimed. "What else?"

Sophie's body pressed hard against mine. "I don't care, Mommy. It doesn't matter what we do."

My babies don't need Fun Mommy, I realized. *They just need Mommy.* I kissed my girlies good night and went to rest in my own bed.

As I drifted off to sleep, I vowed for the hundredth time to fight this beast as hard as I could. *For my girls.*

Although I have two daughters, I like to say I have "one of each." Sophie is Brad's "mini-me." She looks just like pictures of Brad as a child—except for the nose. I don't know where Sophie got her nose. It's elegantly shaped and covered with lovely little freckles.

"If I had your nose," I always tell Sophie, "I could conquer the world."

Sophie is sometimes painfully shy with new people and in new situations. She's a planner. She doesn't like change. While she eats lunch, she asks what's for dinner. She just likes to know what's coming up next.

Sophie makes you earn her love. Whew, that girl's a tough sell. But once it's earned, her love is yours for life. When her best friend ran for the student council in fourth grade, Sophie was ecstatic to serve as her campaign manager. She couldn't have worked any harder on the campaign if she herself had been vying for office. And when her little friend won, Sophie rejoiced.

Sophie's moral compass points steadfastly true north, always. She cannot fathom injustice. She cannot fathom cruelty. She sees only the good, because she doesn't know anything else exists.

Her moral compass points true north
She's fearless though she's scared to death
She makes you earn it, it's worth the wait
She'd never hurt a fly
If I had her heart, the world would be mine,
Who could resist this valentine?
If I had her nose, I could conquer the world
Little freckles, oh so loverly
She's my girl

At the beginning of chemo, I assured Sophie that, thanks to our new baby sitter, her routine wouldn't change at all. "In fact, it might be kind of fun to have someone to play with you all the time, unlike your boring old mom, who's always gotta make dinner or something," I coaxed.

"But I won't be with *you*, Mommy," Sophie said. "I'd rather be with you at home than go to Disneyland with a baby sitter."

Oh, Sophie.

And then there's Chloe, age seven. *My* "mini-me." The anti-Sophie.

Chloe belly flops into the pool of life. She doesn't think about anything but *right this very minute*. For better and for worse. She has not once in her seven years asked me what's for dinner. She doesn't need to know. That's later, and this is now. As if she's a yogini in India, she loves to tell Sophie, "Just be in the moment."

In direct contrast with Sophie, Chloe throws her love around like confetti on New Year's Eve. She throws it up, up, up and away!—and then lets it shimmer down, down, down, dispersing everywhere. She never worries where it might land or that she might run out of it. And, of course, she never runs out. Chloe might be in love with a particular boy today (and she is always googly-eyed over someone), but tomorrow she will find a new love.

Darling Chloe is a ham. More than a ham, actually—so much more: She's a ham-and-cheese sandwich. Chloe would do anything, anything at all, to get a laugh. It's worrisome sometimes, but usually it's just plain funny.

When we were having dinner at a restaurant in Disneyland, Chloe politely excused herself from the table to use the restroom. A few minutes later, she returned and sat quietly back down in her chair.

What a refined young lady! Such manners!

And then Chloe leaned in and whispered to me, totally deadpan, "Winnie the Poop."

I knew I shouldn't laugh. But I did. Bad Mommy! I snorted so loudly, I had to hide my face in my napkin so as not to make a rude commotion in the restaurant. More inappropriate encouragement for the ham-and-cheese-sandwich.

When I picked up Chloe from school one day in second grade, I asked about her day.

"Today was great," she said. "Meditation class was fantastic."

I hadn't been aware that the school offered meditation classes. "You're taking a meditation class?" I asked.

"No, Mom, I'm *teaching* a meditation class."

"Really?" I tried not to laugh. "What do you teach in the class?"

"Oh, you know. Close your eyes. Take a deep breath. Think of a beautiful place." She closed her eyes and breathed in deeply. Then she opened her eyes and shrugged her little shoulders. "Everyone thinks it's really relaxing."

"Who's everyone? How many kids are in this meditation class?"

Her lips moved as she ticked off the names of her pupils to herself. "Eight."

Eight second-graders stood around at recess and followed Guru Chloe in meditation exercises? Whatever happened to hopscotch and tetherball?

I got some dynamite, got a little stick of dynamite
And she gonna go high into the sky
She doesn't walk
She's always dancing down the street
She don't know what's on her balance sheet
She don't care if she's the only one
Doesn't want an entourage, just wants to have some fun

During my weeks and weeks of chemotherapy, as I was forced to spend much of my time in quiet pursuits at home, my girls and I discovered how much we enjoyed each other's company. Sometimes we mulled over a jigsaw puzzle together, chatting the whole time. Other times, they taught me the latest card games they'd learned from their cousins. And sometimes—my favorite times—I'd lift up the corner of my bedspread and say, "Come on in." And the girls and I would nestle in close in my warm bed and watch all six hours of my beloved *Pride and Prejudice*. At the closing credits, Sophie, who'd clearly inherited the period-drama-junkie gene, would beg, "Oh, Mommy! Let's watch it again."

That's my girl!

My Dearest Jane,
What about when Darcy first meets Elizabeth at that ball,
and Elizabeth overhears Mr. Darcy say she is not handsome
enough to tempt him to dance, and then she brazenly walks
past him and gives him the best "F U" look while still smiling.
OMG, I love that part.
XO Laura

Good Morning Laura,
What about when Darcy is tortured by his love/lust for
Elizabeth and he says "I shall conquer this, I shall!" and, even
though Elizabeth is not aware of it, you just think, "For good-
ness' sake, woman, grab him and have him!"
Love, Jane xx

Chapter 41

A few days before my eighth and final chemo infusion, I took Buster to the dog park. I sat on the park bench wearing my head scarf, feeling depleted but happy to be alive under the warm California sun. As I jotted song lyrics in my journal, a man of about fifty entered the gated park with his chocolate Labrador retriever. Buster started jumping for joy at the sight of this other dog, and, once the Lab was unleashed, they galloped off together to play.

The man introduced himself to me as Sal and asked me about Buster. What breed? How old? "He's very handsome," he commented. And then he looked me in the eyes and asked pointedly, "How are you feeling, if you don't mind my asking?" He inquired with such warmth, such genuine caring, that I felt a prickle of a tear forming in my eye.

"Actually, this is my first day out of the house in a full week," I told him honestly. "But I'm feeling okay today."

He didn't ask me if I was a cancer patient; he already knew.

"I've had cancer three times," Sal said gently. "And I had chemo all three times."

He's gone through this three times?!

Sal continued. "Twice, I was given less than a ten percent chance to live. But I never gave up. Ever. When it was hard, I let myself feel that. But I never stayed down for long. I always looked ahead to everything being better. And it always, always got better. It will for you, too."

I was deeply moved. I told him that so much of the time, strangers either ignored me or uttered one of about ten stock platitudes. It had been a long time since I'd struck up a comfortable conversation with a stranger.

Sal laughed and nodded his head. He knew exactly what I was talking about. "Tell me the platitudes."

I rattled them off, counting them on my fingers. "God has a plan. God doesn't give you more than you can handle. Everything happens for a reason. Stay positive." (Mind you, I don't actually disagree with any of these statements, and I understand completely that some people don't know what to say. Still, when you've heard the same exact sentiments, however sincerely meant, from fifty people, it's hard to refrain from checking off a mental box when they're shared.)

It was fun to talk shop with a fellow warrior. It felt sort of . . . taboo to say these things out loud. Liberating. I was on a roll. "The one that actually made me mad," I told Sal, "was 'I know you wouldn't let anything happen to you. You'd never leave your girls.' That one implies that if I were to succumb to cancer, then I didn't care enough about my girls or try hard enough to live. Like, if I were to die, then I was just a bad mother."

Sal chuckled. He understood completely.

I felt unburdened. I couldn't say these horrible, ungrateful things to anyone else, because no one else would understand. And if I said any of this to "civilians," they'd surely second-guess themselves in every future encounter with me. I didn't want to cause any more discomfort around me than I already did.

I asked Sal about his family. He had three living children, he said, but two of his kids had died.

I couldn't believe it. My heart ached with empathetic grief. *The deaths of two children and cancer three times? What was God's plan in that?*

Of course I told Sal how sorry I was. And that he was a shining beacon of hope for me. If he could survive all that life had thrown at him and remain so full of obvious love and warmth, then I could do it, too. Sal was my lifeline that day.

We then settled into talking about our dogs, our loyal and faithful dogs. How they had helped us both get through our treatments. How love transcends language and analysis—it just *is*.

Just as I was telling Sal that Buster had not left my side for five days and nights after every chemo infusion, an older man of about seventy came into the dog park. He released his dog to play with ours and inched over toward our conversation. Since I was wearing my head scarf and talking about chemo, I figured him to be a cancer survivor who wanted to share his story, or maybe offer some encouragement. At any rate, his body language made it clear he wanted to say something to us.

Sal and I greeted him.

"Can I tell you something?" the man said, without preamble.

"Of course," we replied.

"This is the first day I've been able to leave my house for a full week." He held back tears. "My son committed suicide a week ago." His voice was breaking, along with his heart. "I don't know how to survive this."

I touched his shoulder, at a loss for words.

My mind was spinning. Here were three strangers sitting at a dog park one weekday morning in San Diego: a thirtysomething-year-old cancer patient coming down the home stretch of grueling treatment, a seventysomething-year-old man grieving the loss of his child mere days before, and a fiftysomething-year-old man who had survived each of the hardships we were suffering—cancer three times and the death of a child twice. What were the odds?

Sal offered the man heartfelt words of compassion and under-standing, gleaned from his unimaginable similar losses. I saw the man's broken heart soak up Sal's words like a sponge, just as my fragile little heart had soaked up Sal's encouraging comments to me moments before. Sal was this man's lifeline that day, just as he had been mine.

Where was God's plan in that? Right in front of my face.

The day before my eighth and final chemo infusion, just for kicks, I tried putting eyebrow pencil on my bare brow bone (try saying that three times fast). There were about four eyebrow hairs still hanging on to guide my pencil, and I applied the most subtle, color-matching job I could muster. I even used delicate feather strokes, as I'd learned several months earlier at a cancer-themed beauty seminar.

After all this effort, I stood back and looked at myself in the mirror—and then I laughed out loud. I looked ridiculous. Like Carrot Top, the comedian. I got a washcloth and wiped off the eyebrow makeup—only to realize that I had just rubbed off all four of my remaining eyebrow hairs. As I stood in the bathroom all alone, looking at my four eyebrows on this washcloth, I started to belly-laugh. I sat down on the side of the bathtub, laughing and holding my sides. *This is frickin' nuts.*

And just like that, a switch flipped inside me. *I'm done with this.* Of course, I had one final chemo infusion left, and radiation thereafter, but you know what? I wasn't going to let those facts define me. *Hell no.*

I was done deferring to every creak and pain in my body. I was done marking days on a calendar. I was done waiting to reach "the end" of treatment. Life simply could not be solely about *getting through* something—even if that something was chemo or cancer. It had to be about *living.* Life must be lived. Nothing changes that, I realized. Nothing.

It was a glorious spring day—a perfect day for a hike. Brad and I packed the girls into the car for a three-mile hike up a local mountain. With Brad as our fearless leader, the girls and I climbed and climbed, our legs pumping as hard as they would go. It took us over an hour to reach the top, but we were rewarded for our efforts: We could see all the way for miles, into downtown, out to the ocean, and all the way to Mexico. The girls "oohed" and "ahhed" at the view—particularly impressed they could see a whole other country from up there.

From our peak on top of the world, Brad leaned in to me and whispered, "I still love my life; I wouldn't trade it."

He had taken the words right out of my mouth.

I'm not too clever, I'm downright trite
Used to be dark, but now I'm light
Happy to be alive with you,
With you, with you, sweet you
There is no place I'd rather be
Than with you here right now
No place I'd rather be

Nurse Julie unhooked the chemo tube from my port for the eighth and final time, just as two other nurses handed me flowers and tossed confetti over my head. No more chemo smells. No more Barcaloungers. No more nausea. No more . . . feeling poisoned. *No more.*

Brad grabbed my arm, and we marched out of the chemo lounge in triumph. We both knew the hell I'd experience for the next week or so, once the chemo drugs began wreaking havoc on my body. But we also knew another thing: This would be the very last time.

Chapter 42

My next and final stop on the cancer-
treatment train (and Jane's, too): about six weeks of radiation therapy.
Radiation is designed to kill any remaining rogue cells that may have
survived surgery or chemotherapy. Unlike chemotherapy, which is
a systemic treatment (i.e., medicine is introduced into the patient's
blood), radiation is localized, meaning that only the specific areas
where cancer has been found are treated.

Before radiation actually began, doctors plotted the parameters
of my radiation field precisely. As I lay naked from the waist up on a
big metal table, a huge machine out of a sci-fi movie hummed around
me, measuring to within fractions of a millimeter. Precise measure-
ments were critical to ensure proper treatment: Radiating my breast,
chest wall, and armpit? Good. Radiating my heart and lungs? Bad.

While the machine measured, I lay perfectly still for forty-five
minutes, with my arms above my head. After about twenty minutes,
my arms went numb. And then I felt an itch on my face I desperately

wanted to scratch. And then . . . I started to . . . smell something. What was that smell? *Oh, it's me.*

Apparently, my body was aggressively sweating out the remainder of the chemotherapy drugs. (And, unfortunately, wearing deodorant in radiation was prohibited because it somehow interfered with the machines.) It wasn't pretty.

The radiation technician came into the room and sat beside me.

"Please continue to lie very still," he instructed. And then he marked three dots on my body with a Sharpie pen—one dot on my sternum, another one under my breast, and another one under my armpit—the three coordinates of my radiation field.

As the doctor sat next to my armpit, leaning in to do whatever was necessary with that Sharpie pen, I felt self-conscious about my body odor. I figured it was better to acknowledge the elephant in the room than pretend it didn't exist.

"I'm sorry for my stink," I blurted.

The technician smiled at me. "You're fine." And when I didn't say anything, he added, "Remember, we treat other areas of the body here, too." He winked.

Well, I hadn't considered that.

The next step was to permanently tattoo the radiation-field dots to ensure that over the course of the next six weeks, the exact same field on my body would be radiated every time.

Jane had received her radiation tattoos the prior day, and she had emailed to warn me. "Brace yourself, Laura. It hurts terribly."

As the technician raised the tattoo needle in his hand, I steeled myself for the pain. But as the needle pierced my flesh, I didn't even flinch.

"Wow," the technician said. "Most people say that really hurts."

I guess most people aren't She-Ra, Princess of Power. "Oh, that's nothing," I scoffed. "Pfft." During the second and third tattoos, I could have fallen asleep.

Nothing to it!

Just like that, I was now the tattooed lady. Granted, the tattoos were eensy-weensy, barely visible, but I knew they were there. (And, by the way, the moment I got home from the hospital, I emailed Jane to tell her that she was a "complete and total wuss.") And the coolest thing? My radiation tattoos had "broken the seal," so to speak. I would never go back to my tattooless self.

Well, I thought, *I might as well get a real one now. Let the permanent badassery begin!*

Over the next six weeks, I went in for radiation treatments five times per week. Every day I lay down on the big metal table and R2-D2 buzzed around me, radiating the three areas designated by my radiation tattoos. *Zap. Zap. Zap.* Getting undressed and into my hospital gown took longer than the actual radiation session.

Radiation reminded me of something Sharon said right after her triplets were born. Her husband had taken their older daughter out for an entire afternoon of entertainment, leaving Sharon at home alone with their three infants, and Sharon gushed to me, in sincere relief, "Gosh, it's so much easier to care for three kids than four."

For me, radiation was like caring for twins (pun intended) after having served a long tour of duty with quintuplets. A virtual vacation.

True, there were side effects as the long weeks of daily treatments took their toll on my body. The biggest was what the doctors called "fatigue." And it was certainly true that I fell asleep the moment my head hit the pillow every night. Occasionally I napped, too. But you know what? *Fatigue shmatigue.*

True, my radiated skin became blistered and pained. And toward the end, it tightened like leather. But, at least for me, this problem did not compare to months of chemotherapy. The superficial pain from radiation was isolated within my breast, chest, and armpit; it did not touch my heart, mind, and soul. My spirit remained untethered from my circumstances.

It wasn't long before downy-soft hairs started sprouting on my scalp. I was reborn. Brad couldn't keep his hands off my newborn head. He constantly rubbed it and called my little hairlings "beautiful."

Unfortunately, the hair follicles in my scalp were not the only ones becoming active again. In addition to the beautiful hair on my head, I was developing noticeable peach fuzz all over my entire face.

"You've got muttonchops," Brad teased, and I promptly bee-lined to the bathroom to shave my cheeks with his electric razor. (Thankfully, the peach fuzz subsided after a few weeks.)

I started going to weekly Pilates classes, where my classmates took great interest in tracking the progress of my hair growth from week to week. I took daily walks with Buster. I started, very slowly, to see my friends again.

And then, toward the end of my radiation treatments, I sang with Cool Band Luke at a fundraising gala for lung cancer. My hair was at the G.I. Jane stage, so I wore a red flapper wig throughout the performance. I shook my booty all night long, and no one ever suspected I was in the midst of cancer treatments. I was just the girl in the band. It felt like coming home.

At the end of the night, after the lights had come on and the band was packing up our gear, I took off the wig, which had become hot and itchy. A lingering partygoer gasped when I removed it and exclaimed, "You look better without the wig! Ditch the wig!"

Thanks to that kind (or drunk) stranger, I donated the wig and all my head scarves to a cancer charity the very next day and never covered up again.

A few weeks later, my head was sprouting a curly mop. And though I was grateful to have hair at all, this Q-tip look wasn't particularly attractive. "I look like Vinny Barbarino from *Welcome Back, Kotter*," I whined to Brad.

"Oh, no, you don't, honey," Brad reassured me. And just as I was about to hug him, he added, "You look like Horshack."

But nothing could get me down. I had hair again. My port had been removed. I had no nausea or bone pain. We had (gratefully) said goodbye to our (wonderful) baby sitter. It was time for our family to take care of itself again.

And then, like a faucet that has suddenly been turned on, new songs started pouring into my head. They flooded me at all times of the day and night, boring holes through my gray matter.

I was back, baby! There was no doubt about it.

Chapter 43

Jane and I were engaged in an enthusiastic email exchange about how to cast the movie about our lives. I definitely wanted Julia Roberts or Sandra Bullock to play me, or, if the movie included a younger me, maybe Anne Hathaway. Any of them would do, really; I loved them all. (Not very original, I know, but you've got to aim for the top.)

"At any rate," I reasoned, ever the pragmatist, "I'd need an A-list actress to play me to get the project green-lit." I was proud of myself for using such in-the-know industry-speak.

Jane agreed that my entertainment-industry acumen was admirable. "For me," she joined in, "it's got to be Cate Blanchett or Renée Zellweger. Either of them would do me justice."

"I understand Cate," I responded, having established myself as the resident Hollywood expert, "but Renée Zellweger to play *you*? An *American*? Perish the thought!"

"Oh, yes," Jane shot back. "Renée did a bang-up British accent in the Bridget Jones movies."

Actually, I'd read an article in which Hugh Grant had said Renée's accent had been impeccable. Perhaps Jane was onto something there. "Good point, Jane." Really, we'd missed our mutual callings. We both should have been Hollywood casting agents. "So hard to choose." (And, of course, it was imperative we make a decision soon, since Hollywood was sure to be knocking down our doors any day now.)

"What about Brad?" Jane asked.

"That's easy," I wrote. "Brad Pitt will play my Brad. Brad Pitt's a dead ringer for his irreverence and charm." And, I recalled, the two Brads had been members of the same fraternity at their respective colleges. That being the case, my Brad and Angelina's Brad (or dare I call him "Angie's Brad"?) could greet each other on the movie set with secret handshakes and sappy fraternity songs—about which Angie and I would roll our eyes and exchange warm looks of commiseration about our beloved men. *They're so silly,* our mutual expressions would communicate, *but oh, how we love them.*

And now that I thought about it, if Angelina Jolie wanted to star in my movie with her Brad, then I most certainly would not stand in her way. It had been an egregious oversight to overlook her as a candidate to play me in the first place, I realized. I wasn't totally convinced she could pull off my particular brand of spazziness—she seemed like a pretty cool customer to me—but I would be open to letting her try.

"Well then," Jane wrote, and I could detect her bossy tone clearly through cyberspace, across two continents, "how about a cute boyfriend for me? I'd like Hugh Jackman, please," she commanded, as if she were ordering fish and chips. "That man can sing! You could do a duet with him in the movie, maybe in a dream sequence or something."

It made no sense! Jane was unattached at the moment! And this movie was meant to be cinema verité—as realistic and gritty as possible.

Ha! Who was I kidding? If my Brad and I were Brad Pitt and Angelina Jolie, then by God, My Dearest Jane would enjoy a torrid, if fantastical, affair with Hugh Jackman. It was our movie, wasn't it?

"Okay, Jane. We'll create a part for Hugh Jackman." I laughed as I pressed the "send" button. It was the least I could do for my dear friend.

Come to think of it, that gave me an idea: As long as we were creating parts that made absolutely no sense in this movie, couldn't we find a part for George Clooney (twice honored as *People* magazine's Sexiest Man Alive, if you haven't heard)? Given George's years of experience portraying a TV doctor on *ER*, perhaps he could be Dr. Hampshire in our film.

"George is my absolute favorite!" I wrote.

"Oh, yes, he's a dream," Jane replied.

"He's such a man's man, isn't he?" I sighed. "I bet he smells like Old Spice! I just want to get right up close and . . . smell him."

During those interminable months of chemo, my sense of smell had become particularly acute as the unmistakable and omnipresent odors of chemicals and sickness had bombarded my nostrils. I just hadn't been able to escape that awful chemo scent, though I'd changed my sheets and pajamas obsessively—it was on my skin, my clothes, my sheets.

Yes, I decided, George Clooney's manly-man smell would be an idyllic escape from cancer and its wafting stranglehold on my life. Yes, George Clooney's Old Spice smell would be just the ticket to take me away from it all.

"Oh, Laura," Jane wrote in her reply email, "is he your celebrity crush? The one you'd 'do' if given the chance?"

"I don't want to have *sex* with him, Jane," I wrote piously, though, of course, I was lying. "I just want to smell him!"

I just want this to be over.

For the hundredth time, I thought about my bucket list, something I'd composed in my mind, and supplemented many times, as I'd lain in bed on my darkest days. Some of the items on the list were meaningful and poignant, exactly as you'd expect. Like watching my daughters graduate from college. Or holding my future grandchildren in my arms. Or taking golf lessons so I could join Brad on the course in our twilight years.

But life is also about moments of giddy excitement, flashes of unexpected, pulse-racing thrill. Isn't it?

Yes, the more I thought about my bucket list, the more I realized smelling George Clooney was pretty high on the list. And, dammit, I wasn't ashamed to admit it.

I want to be the kind of girl who eats sushi and has tattoos
Always a witty comeback, drinkin' gin and vermouth
I want to sing my songs in Prague and wear a coat in London fog
Go down to 'Nawlins on the Dog, never sit at a desk job
I wanna laugh and sing all day, thinking's purely optional

I've thought a lot, I'm done with that, and now I'm having fun
I wanna smell George Clooney
I bet he'd smell real good
I'd wrap my arms around him
And I would breathe him in
Yeah, I would breathe him in
I want my "happy" and my "right,"
I won't give up without a fight
I want to see my name in lights
It's finite, my dear
Life is finite, my dear

When I emerged from my very last radiation treatment and into the hospital waiting room, my fellow radiation patients, whom I had befriended over the past several weeks of daily treatments, threw me a "radiation graduation party." My song "Mama Needs a Girls' Night Out" was blaring on the CD player, and we all started dancing around in our hospital gowns, booties hanging out and all. After cake and presents and warm hugs all around, I walked out of the radiation area as the group hummed "Pomp and Circumstance."

Brad and I marched out the front doors of the hospital together, arm in arm, and at the first flash of bright sunshine on my face, I raised my arms in triumph. We'd reached the finish line.

Before heading to the car, though, we made one last stop, in the building next door.

"Sayonara," I said to Dr. Hampshire, real sassy-like, as I stood in his office.

"You're not nearly done with me," he reminded me. (Indeed, regular checkups with my oncologist would be part of my life for years to come.)

"I know," I admitted. "But it feels so good to say that today. Just humor me, Doc. *Sayonara!*"

Brad and I drove to an artsy area of town for a celebratory lunch at an outdoor Italian café. We basked in the San Diego sunshine and smiled at each other until our cheeks hurt. *It's over.*

"Babe, I want to get a tattoo," I announced over my seafood pasta.

Brad paused for just a moment, smirking at me in his usual "oh, Lucy" sort of way. "Of what?"

I told him.

"Honey," Brad began, the voice of reason, "a tattoo may seem like a great idea *now*. But one day you'll be old and saggy and you'll totally regret it."

I considered what he had said for a moment. It was a relief to note that he had reverted to assuming I'd live to old age—a welcome change from his despair of only a few months before.

"The way I see it, I can't lose. Either I get a tattoo and love it for the rest of my life, however long or short that is, or I live long enough to regret it one day. I'd love to live long enough to regret a tattoo."

Brad laughed. "You make a great point." He shook his head as if shaking off a bad dream. "I can't argue with that logic."

Brad paid the bill and we ran, holding hands, to the tattoo parlor across the street, where I told the tattoo artist the phrase I wanted him to "ink" on my body. (I'm sure I didn't actually use the word "ink" at the time, but in the retelling, it makes me seem edgier, doesn't it?)

"What font do you want for the letters?" the tattoo artist asked me.

I hadn't thought about that. "I have no idea."

He referred me to a computer with hundreds of fonts, each identified by name.

"Just take a look through all of these and let me know which one you want," he said, and turned to walk away, apparently assuming this was going to take a while.

I squinted down at the list of fonts. How on earth was I going to pick from so many options? I started scanning.

Bingo. Third one down from the top. I didn't need to look any further.

"Okay!" I called to the tattoo artist, summoning him back. He hadn't even made it out of the room yet. "I found it." I pointed. "*That one.*"

"Sounds good. Lie down here," he said, motioning to an adjacent table.

I complied.

The tattoo guy prepared his instruments and explained the process to me.

I pulled up my shirt, unhooked the clasp of my bra, and positioned my body on its right side, beaming at Brad the whole time.

Brad watched in total fascination as the tattoo artist carefully inscribed—in Jane Austen font, of course!—the phrase "I'm still here" next to my scarred and embattled breast, just under my left armpit.

I'm still here!

Not too long ago, when I'd inhaled pot for the first time, I'd hung up my goody-two-shoes for good. And now, with each plunge of the tattoo needle into my skin, I was donating those damned shoes to the Salvation Army.

Oh yeah, sucka? How ya like me now? I'm still here!

I kicked you hard and I'm not sorry,
I beat you up and it felt good
Said hit the road, Jack, and I meant it
With half a chance, I'd do it again
Kiss-off of the century,
Slamming the door on your back as you leave
Don't come back, don't come back, don't you never come back!
Just the beginning of me
Get out! Stay out! Time's out! And I'm starting all over
Stand out! Rock out! Break out! I'm my own superhero
Nothing to pout about, just gotta shout about: I'm still here!
Nothing to pout about, just gotta shout about: I'm still here!

When we returned home from our eventful afternoon, I showered the girls with confetti. And though Sophie was appalled by my new tattoo ("How *could* you?"), all was forgiven in her relief to have her mommy back.

"Oooh, I love your tattoo, Mommy," Chloe purred, in direct contrast with Sophie's horrified reaction. I could see her eyes light up, even at age seven, with what she perceived to be my implicit approval of her future, teenage tattoo.

"You know," I told Chloe, "I waited to get a tattoo until I was thirty-eight and had kicked cancer's booty."

Yeah, yeah, Chloe's mischievous eyes said to me. *Blah blah blah.*

A few days later, I picked up the girls from school for the first time in many months. Because I had been in treatment for so long, their classmates had not seen me with any regularity during the school year, and they didn't know me. As I waited outside Sophie's third-grade classroom, one of her classmates, Josephine, emerged first.

"Whose mommy are you?" Josephine asked me.

"I'm Sophie's mommy."

"Oh, yeah, I know you. I didn't know you cut your hair." She sounded so mature.

"Well, actually, I didn't cut my hair. It came out because of some medicine I took, but now it's growing back."

The look on her face told me she'd already heard about what had been happening to Sophie's mommy. "I'm glad you didn't die," she said matter-of-factly.

"Me too."

My Dearest Jane,

We have been hand in hand, our legs tied together in a three-legged race, and now we have hurtled across the finish line together! And this summer, when I come to the UK for my music, we will hug, and drink a "pint," and laugh and laugh and laugh together at our stubbly little heads and the amazing journey we have traveled together!

XOXO Laura

Chapter 44

The first six months following my cancer treatments were a whirlwind of activity, despite Brad's constant admonishments to me to "take it easy." I was making up for lost time—trying to prove to myself, and everyone else, that I was "back."

The first item on my agenda? My "Laura Kicked Cancer's Ass" comeback concert at a renowned local venue called the Belly Up. That night was like attending my own funeral, without the death part. The place was packed to the rafters with family, friends, fans of the *Jeff & Jer* show, fellow cancer survivors, and, much to my delight, the doctors and nurses who'd saved my life.

Before the Laura Roppé Band hit the stage, we smashed our bodies into a group hug backstage, energized by the expectant hum of the waiting crowd.

"I love you guys!" I shouted into the huddle, above the din.

"We love you, too, Laura!" came the energetic reply.

Out in the club, the hum was becoming a roar.

"Let's do it!" I whooped to my band.

"Hell yeah!" is what came back.

As my band made its way onto the stage, joined by my cousin Matthew as our guest guitarist for the night, I remained backstage momentarily. I could feel a tidal wave of anticipation fill the club. *Is she there? Where is she?*

Grinning from ear to ear, I climbed the back steps of the stage and walked down to front and center. A tsunami of love crashed onto the stage and flooded all the way up to the rafters of the joint. The roar in that crowded club was deafening.

When my drummer counted off "one . . . two . . . three . . . four!" the band launched into a rousing version of "Girl Like This," and the crowd exploded. We were off to the races! And though I had not originally considered myself the girl in that song, in that moment, there was no doubt that, at least for that night, I was the rare girl with "magic in her fingertips."

After several high-energy songs to get the crowd going, the lights dimmed and Matthew joined me at the front of the stage on a stool, his acoustic guitar at the ready. I smiled at him, and then I turned back to the crowd.

"When I was little, I needed a 'woobie' to keep me safe from nightmares." I shielded my eyes from the bright stage lights and, after a brief moment of searching the crowd, found Brad's handsome face, a head taller than most people around him, in the audience. "During the nightmare of this past year, my husband, Brad, was my woobie."

You could hear a pin drop in the crowd. I continued, looking into Brad's blue eyes, "This song is for you, babe."

Matt began playing his guitar and I started to sing "Woobie," the song inspired by Brad's heartbreaking cries in his sleep, for which Matt had composed a heartfelt guitar accompaniment:

> *Don't cry, it'll be all right*
> *I'll be your woobie, hold on to me tight*
> *Baby, baby, you're my woobie*
> *Baby, baby, I'm yours, too*
> *I don't want no other woobie*
> *Baby, all I want is you*
>
> *Baby, all I want is you.*

Brad had journeyed every step of the way with me through the fires of hell. He had shielded me as best he could as I'd walked through the flames, and then he'd lovingly wrapped bandages around my burns and battle scars. And Matt, my beloved cousin, now playing his guitar so beautifully, had willingly jumped onto my tour bus to Hades, right into the seat next to mine, and had strummed his guitar as a means of distracting me from the horrific view out the window. It was a magical moment for the three of us.

It was the official end of my tour of duty as a cancer patient.

After the girls and I, like summer campers on uppers, had methodically ticked off every entry on our When Mommy Gets

Better To-Do List—Sea World! The beach! The pool! Duck feeding! A picnic!—I giddily boarded a London-bound airplane in August 2009. My mission? Cross off two items on my bucket list: (1) filming the much-anticipated music video for "Float Away"—the carrot that had been dangling in front of my face since the moment I'd been diagnosed—and (2) drinking a "pint" with My Dearest Jane, the honorary sister who had held my hand, from across the pond, throughout my whole ordeal.

When I exited customs at Heathrow Airport, a gentleman was standing in the waiting crowd with a sign that read Ms. ROPPÉ. I'd always wanted to be one of those passengers whose name was written on a sign at the airport. He'd even gotten the accent on the *é* right!

The gentleman was a very proper British man with a fancy car (whose steering wheel had been placed on the wrong side of the car; someone had neglected to tell him). John from London had sent this gentleman to "collect me" at the airport. It was all so very "posh."

On the drive to the hotel, the gentleman asked me what I was doing in the UK.

"I'm here to shoot a music video," I replied. Ha! I sounded like I was making that up. *Yes, I'm here to shoot a music video. And to take tea and crumpets with the Queen.* Both statements sounded equivalently preposterous to me. But the former was true!

"Oh, so you're a singer, are you?" the gentleman asked.

"Yes, I am." *And I'm in London! To shoot a music video!*

At my hotel in the heart of Kensington, a swanky area of London, I asked the front desk if Jane had checked in yet. She would be coming in on the train, Jane had said, and would meet me at the hotel around the time of my arrival from the airport.

The front-desk clerk checked the computer. "Not yet, madam."

"Well, please, the moment she checks in, will you give her my room number and ask her to call me there?" I rushed through my words like an excited three-year-old.

My room turned out to be an airy suite overlooking the city. There was a fruit basket on the coffee table. I had always wished for a fruit basket in a hotel room. I looked out the window and marveled at the view. I unpacked my clothes. I sat on the bed, staring at the phone. I ate some of the fruit. I jumped in the shower.

Just as I turned on the water, the phone rang.

I jumped out of the shower and dashed to the phone.

"Jane!" I answered loudly.

"Laura!" came the effusive reply. There were hysterical giggles on both sides. It was the first time we pen pals had heard each other's flesh–and–blood voices.

"Where are you?" I shouted, unable to speak at normal levels.

"Fourth floor!"

"Stay put! I'm coming, Jane!" I threw my clothes back on as if I'd been jolted by a fire alarm, and then I sprinted out my hotel room and down the common hallway to the elevator at the end of the hall. I pressed the call button for the elevator, rocking back and forth in nervous anticipation. When the doors opened, I jumped inside and repeatedly punched the button to the fourth floor as the doors closed.

Was this the slowest elevator in the world?

Ding! The elevator doors opened, and I wanted to dart out at full throttle! But there were two hallways extending out from opposite sides of the elevator. I wasn't sure which way to go.

"Jane!" I hollered, peeking my head outside the elevator doors.

"Laura!" came a voice to my left. I ran, following the voice.

And then there she was at the end of the hallway, a beaming smile on her face: My Dearest Jane.

I barreled toward Jane and she hurtled toward me until we collided in the middle, hugging each other and laughing uncontrollably. We hugged and hugged, tears streaming down our cheeks. After we had pulled away to look at each other's beautiful, glowing faces, we hugged again.

I pulled back to get a good look at My Dearest Jane. She was about five inches shorter than I am, with light hair and crystal blue eyes. She was my physical opposite in every way, except for one thing: We shared identical fuzzy crew cuts.

I ran my hand across her baby-soft hair, and she returned the favor.

"Oh, Jane!" I laughed. "We're twins!"

Back in Jane's hotel room, I met her blast-from-the-past boyfriend, David. Jane and David had known, and loved, each other as young children in Sheffield. When David's family had moved away, he and Jane had lost touch and their love story had ended.

Or so they'd thought. Thirty years later, just a few months before my visit, David had rediscovered the sassy girl from his childhood on Facebook. And, unaware that Jane had been married and recently separated from her husband, or that she had a two-year-old daughter, or that she was in the middle of chemotherapy for triple negative breast cancer, he had invited her to dinner.

Of course, David had found out soon enough about Jane's industrial-size baggage when she'd shown up for dinner in a head scarf and vanishing eyebrows. But guess what? None of that mattered. David could see *Jane*—not just her stupid container. From that very first dinner, they had become inseparable, baggage and all.

For the first three days of my trip, Jane, David, and I painted London Town red. We went to see famed palaces, feeding our mutual love of Henry VIII and his six wives (do you think I'm weird?); we toured museums; we went to parks and pubs (where Jane and I finally sat down to drink that pint together); we ate gluttonous meals, including a full-blown Mexican feast in honor of my beloved San Diego, so many thousands of miles away (oddly enough, my tacos were pretty good).

And, best of all, we went to a karaoke piano bar.

The small bar was crammed with young people from wall to wall, singing along with abandon as the piano man played songs from Kings of Leon to Elton John. After a few Peroni beers, I enthusiastically joined the sing-along, arm in arm with Jane: "You know that I could use somebody . . . someone like youuuuu!"

Occasionally, a bar patron sang into the piano man's mic, leading the raucous crowd in song. After several songs, Jane nudged my shoulder gently toward the piano, saying, "Go on, Laura, go on. Sing." But no one had to twist my arm.

I asked the piano man, "Do you know 'Waterfalls,' by TLC?"

"Sure," he said. "What key?"

I told him and then addressed the crowd in full Cool Band Luke mode: "Hey, everyone! I bring you greetings all the way from San Diego, Californiaaaa!" The bar erupted. When I launched into the song—"a lonely mother gazin' out of her window, starin' at a son that she just can't touch . . . "—the crowd went "mad" (as they say in Britain). The energy in the bar from the start of the song was off the charts, but when I got to the hardcore rap in the middle, the roof blew off the place. People started jumping up and down and hugging each other, as if England had just won the World Cup. At the end of the song, the entire bar started chanting, "USA! USA!" Strangers kissed my cheeks and lifted me up off the floor.

Blame it on the free-flowing beer, or maybe on my "exotic" American accent, but something magical happened in that bar that night. Maybe they could feel my sheer joy at being alive. Or at being able to sing again. Or maybe, just maybe, they really, really liked "Waterfalls." (It's a great groove, after all.) All I know is, on that particular evening, a horde of Brits crowded around a piano in a cramped bar and sent unadulterated love to the happy American girl with the very short hair. And she sent it right back to each and every one of them.

The next morning, it was time to say goodbye to Jane. I was emotional. We had held each other's hands through cyberspace for months and months, through the darkest time in both of our lives. Being able to finally touch Jane, and hug her, and hear the sound of her voice, had been an unforgettable gift. And now, after so short a time, we had to say goodbye.

"Don't worry," Jane comforted me, "this won't be the last you see of me."

Chapter 45

Just as Jane and David left London to go back home, my violinist, Jennifer, arrived. From our first chance meeting online, just over a year before, through band rehearsals, performances, and recording on my album, to endless conversations, emails, and visits during my cancer treatments, Jennifer had become one of my dearest friends. Since she had played violin on "Float Away," it was only fitting that she be featured in the music video, too. And now here she was, her hair braided like Laura Ingalls Wilder and her violin strapped to her back. Adorable.

Moments later, John from London arrived at the hotel with the music video director and some key members of the video crew. (Oh, yes, I said "crew.") The two-day shoot was scheduled to start the next day; today would be all about planning and scheduling.

I had already met John one year earlier, when he'd flown to San Diego to watch my band open for Little Feat, a rock band with a diehard following, mere days before the start of my chemo. The show had been scheduled for months, and despite my intervening diagnosis and then-imminent treatment, I had remained hell-bent on having one last musical hurrah.

It was also the night before I cut off my long hair at the salon. As I sat in the green room before the show with my bandmates, everyone else chatted and laughed, excited about opening for such a popular band. I tried to seem lighthearted and ready to rock, but in reality, my mind was focused on the overwhelming battle that yawned before me.

Onstage, my band performed like the pros they were, but I forgot lyrics to my own songs—my worst nightmare—and wound up repeating the same verses two and three times. And, as Brad told me later, I also swung my long hair around the stage all night like a headbanger—just like the object of my then-recent scorn, Rico Suave—perhaps subconsciously giving it one last ride at the rodeo.

After the show, John came backstage, full of praise. "Well done," he said, in typical British fashion. "Well done. 'Float Away' is what won them over," he observed. "Everyone loves a ballad."

That did seem to be the consensus. Despite what I had considered a poor performance on my part, we had gotten a standing ovation from the crowd, including from Little Feat fans who'd initially had zero interest in seeing us perform. After the show, several of them had approached me to say, "You're my new favorite band—next to Little Feat, of course!"

At least I'm going out with a bang, I thought. And then, for just a moment, this thought flitted across my mind: *Please don't let this be my last performance.*

And now here I was, not even a full year later, giving John from London a big hug in his hometown, as if the prior year had never happened.

"Laura, this is Steve Graham," John said now, motioning to the man next to him. "Our fearless music video director."

But I knew exactly who Steve was. His credits included music videos for the Eurythmics, Lenny Kravitz, Oasis, and Paul McCartney. When John had first told me Steve would be directing my video, I had pinched myself.

"Nice to meet you, Steve," I said calmly, shaking his hand. But on the inside, I was flipping out in typical Laura fashion.

Immediately, Steve opened his laptop and began detailing the locations and logistics of the shoot. He was all business.

I tried to "act like I'd been there before," nodding and smiling—but not too energetically—at everything he was telling me. But when he mentioned that his "crew" had acquired the "permits" for such-and-such "location," I felt like one of my crazy beads had shaken loose and was rolling around inside my head.

The next day, John drove Jenny and me down to Brighton, on England's south coast, for our first day of shooting. Immediately after a brief introduction to my music video family—professional actors hired to play my beleaguered husband and cute-as-a-button daughter—we began filming. It had been many years since my UCLA theater days, and I was nervous.

In my first scene, I cuddled on the beach with my "husband" (an actor named Mark), watching our little "daughter" (a beautiful six-year-old named Billie) as she frolicked on the beach. Cuddling with

Mark before I'd had a chance to get to know him was, admittedly, a bit awkward. But I just tried to imagine he was Brad.

There wasn't any awkwardness with my "daughter," Billie, though. Right away, she crawled into my lap and snuggled close. Her Mary Poppins accent (on a child!) enchanted me, and my American movie-star accent seemed mesmerizing to her. We were like two peas in a pod. It was easy to project my love for Sophie and Chloe onto Billie.

When it was time for Jennifer to play her violin, Billie and I held hands on the sidelines, watching Jenn play under a gazebo overlooking the sea, as the cameras rolled. After the scene, Billie and I and the rest of the cast and crew—as well as a few Brightonites who'd stopped to watch—applauded.

Later in the day, our group moved to a flat that had been rented as a stand-in for my fake family's home. After filming a mock birthday party for Billie—during which the candles on her cake melted away more quickly than anyone had anticipated—Steve suggested we shoot a scene in which Mark and I had a "row."

"Sounds fun," I answered, enjoying every moment.

"What are we fighting about?" Mark asked me.

"I'm neglecting Billie, the housework, you," I suggested. "You want to know what the hell's wrong with me. I've exhausted your patience."

"Brilliant."

Mark and I then proceeded to scream at each other, blaming each other for everything from the laundry on the floor to the demise of our marriage, while the cameras rolled. *Easy peasy!*

But then Steve said it was time to film a scene depicting my spiral into despair. I had been dreading this—not because I couldn't tap into dark emotions, but because I *could*. All too well.

"Do you think you can cry in this scene?" Steve wondered.

Does Dorothy follow the Yellow Brick Road?

"Without a doubt."

When Steve yelled, "Action," I let horrible thoughts creep into my mind: *What if the cancer comes back? What if I have to leave my babies? What if the chemo didn't work?* My tears flowed. I didn't want to give those thoughts entry into my mind, not even for a music video. But, damn, I didn't know how else to cry on demand. Luckily, Steve was thrilled with the scene on the first take and I was free to banish those dark thoughts to the abyss forevermore.

The next day, we left Brighton for Beachy Head in Eastbourne, East Sussex, a site of towering, stunning white cliffs overlooking the magnificent blue ocean. I was told that this was a favorite suicide spot, and I could see why: Despite vertigo-inducing heights, there were no guard rails or warning signs keeping people away from the staggering cliff edges. It was mind boggling, really, to see those plunging cliffs, fully accessible to anyone—so unlike in America, where any accident provokes a lawsuit.

On this day, we were slated to shoot the "performance" scenes in the video—that is, the scenes of me singing along to my song. There would be no other actors or props; the scenes' success would depend on my ability to convey the emotions of my song authentically.

The crew set up canned lighting and guide tracks for the cameras to glide along smoothly, the makeup artist painted my face, and Steve bobbed around, searching for the best angles for his shots. As we waited, John, Jenny, and I sat in the foldable directors' chairs typically seen on movie sets. It was a full-scale production.

A crowd had started to gather to watch the impending filming. *Who is she? I don't recognize her, do you?*

How exciting for them if I had been someone famous!

Sorry, folks, I thought. *It's just me.*

Shooting began. As the camera filmed from a variety of angles, I stood in a fluttery white nightgown at the edge of the steep cliff (but not dangerously close, believe me) and sang along to a recording of "Float Away." After the first run-through of the song, a crew member named Grahame—a muscle-clad bald guy in dark sunglasses, whose job it was to hold a reflector board that bounced light directly onto my face—set down his board and bear-hugged me.

"I'm honored to be here to witness this," Grahame said (although, since he is British, I am sure he was "honoured").

Perhaps due to his manly physique, or maybe his Monty Python accent, I wasn't sure if he was serious. So I asked him, "Are you serious?"

Without a word, Grahame tilted up his sunglasses to reveal big, soggy tears streaming out of his eyes. And then he hugged me again. I couldn't speak. *Really?* I was deeply moved.

Now that we'd wrapped the music video shoot, it was time for a two-week, whirlwind radio tour at BBC radio stations all over the country—London! Manchester! Liverpool! Sheffield! Wales!

One day, John's promotions manager, Harriet, brought me to the BBC radio station in London for a round of interviews. Just as we headed into the station, Harriet whispered, "Oh, there's Wogan's producer." And sure enough, there was Alan Boyd, producer of the *Wake Up to Wogan* radio programme (British spelling, I can't help it), the most listened-to radio show in the entire country. With a draw of eight million loyal listeners every day, airplay on *Wake Up to Wogan* was the holy grail for an artist striving to break into the UK radio market. And the man who decided which songs would air on the Holy Grail—Alan Boyd—was standing a mere ten feet away from me.

As we approached, Mr. Boyd stood outside the front doors of the station, smoking a cigarette (or "smoking a fag.")

Harriet greeted Mr. Boyd and introduced me.

"Oh, yes," Mr. Boyd said. "I've heard your song. I've been intending to play that one. We'll get you on straight away."

I was so elated, I lunged at him, hugged him, and kissed him hard on the cheek, exuberantly invading his personal space. It was a remarkably un-British, and quite American, thing to do. Thankfully, though, Mr. Boyd didn't seem the least bit upset.

"Well done, you," Harriet whispered as we walked away.

Inside the station, Jennifer and I bounced around from studio to studio for interviews and live performances on various radio stations across the country. After one such interview, as Harriet, Jenny, and I walked down a hallway toward the next studio, we passed Mr. Boyd, who was shuffling busily in the opposite direction.

"Hi again," I said cheerfully as we passed each other, but my eyes said, *Please don't forget to play my song!*

"Hello again," he humored me. ("Humoured" me.)

About two hours later, we'd finished all our business at the radio station that day, and we made our way along the street toward the subway ("the Tube"). And, yet again, there was our poor stalking victim, Mr. Boyd, sitting at an outdoor café next to the busy sidewalk.

"Hi again," I said, a bit apologetically, as we passed.

This time, Mr. Boyd called Harriet over to him.

She bent down to hear him speak amid the noisy street traffic. They engaged in a brief conversation as Jenny and I looked on from a short distance away.

"Thank you!" Harriet sang as she walked back toward Jenny and me.

We took a few silent steps to get out of earshot of Mr. Boyd, and then Harriet stage-whispered, "Well done. He says he'll play 'Float Away' tomorrow morning at nine o'clock."

Jenny and I erupted in squeals. We were eleven-year-olds at a Justin Bieber concert.

"Let's just see if he actually comes through," Harriet cautioned.

The next morning, Jennifer and I tuned in to BBC Radio 2's *Wake Up to Wogan* in our hotel room, holding our breath. At the nine o'clock hour, we heard Sir Wogan introduce "a new song from superstar Laura Roppé," followed by the familiar sounds of Jenny's violin progression, leading in to my familiar voice. "She says I think I'll go home, turn off the telephone . . . ," I heard myself sing—to eight million people!

Jenny and I jumped on the hotel beds for joy and danced around the room. Eight million people had just heard my song! It was unfathomable to me. We couldn't enjoy the moment for too long, though, because Harriet was awaiting us downstairs in the lobby for yet another round of radio interviews.

It is such hard work being a "superstar"!

When we met up with Harriet in the lobby, Jenny and I tackled her from both sides. "Did you hear it?! Did you hear it?!"

"Yes," Harriet beamed. "Wonderful news."

That afternoon, John "liaised" with Jenny, Harriet, and me for afternoon tea at Harrods, a very "posh" and famous thing to do in London. The tea was sublime, served with silver spoons and exquisite china, and the biscuits and scones were melt-in-your-mouth delicious. I felt like Queen Elizabeth herself.

"Here's to Wogan," John toasted.

"Here, here."

The next day, John drove Jenny and me to Manchester, one of the biggest and most respected radio markets in the UK, for another interview. *Oh, such hard, hard work!* When I returned to my hotel twelve hours later, having endured hours of snarled traffic to and from Manchester—plus a shopping spree during which I had bought Brad a Manchester United jersey so he could wear it while happily playing his favorite (stupid) soccer video game with our friend Mike—all I wanted to do was sleep. I shuffled through the hotel lobby and dragged myself into the elevator to go back to my room.

Standing in the elevator was an African American man. Over the past few weeks in London, an exceedingly international city, I had grown accustomed to seeing people of every race, creed, and color, and from every continent on the planet, including Africa. But this man was not from Africa, I was certain; I would have bet dollars to doughnuts he was an American.

"Hi," I greeted him as I entered the elevator. My tone was warm.

"Hey," he replied, returning my warmth. *I knew it. American. My countryman!*

"How's it going?"

"Exhausting," he answered.

"Me, too. You want to compare?"

"Sure. You first."

Prepare to be dazzled, my American friend.

"Well," I began, fake boredom in my voice. "I just went all the way to Manchester today for a radio interview. We hit tons of traffic; it took us hours to get there. I had, like, one second to spare when we finally arrived before I had to go live on-air. And then we drove back, again in traffic for hours. Long day."

I know, pretty impressive. I'm sure you're wondering who the hell I am right about now. I considered squeezing in the fact that my song had just aired on *Wake Up to Wogan*, but I couldn't figure out how to shoehorn that into the three-second conversation. Oh well. I was sure he was adequately impressed nonetheless. "Okay, your turn."

We had arrived at the guy's hotel floor. The elevator doors opened, but he stood between the doors, holding them open.

"I'll give you the win for today," he said, "but this tour's been brutal for months."

Tour? "What tour?"

He reached down to grab a laminated credential card on his belt.

He tilted it up to me. "I'm managing U2's world tour." And with that, he hopped off the elevator to the other side of the closing doors.

Just as the doors closed, I shouted to him, smiling, "You win!"

The last sight I saw before the elevator doors closed was the cocky smile on his handsome face. He'd known all along he'd win our contest hands down.

I laughed for a good long time to myself about that one. It served me right.

When it was time to leave the UK, John sent that elegant driver from the first day to "collect" me from my hotel and take me to the airport. When we got there, he wished me safe travels and I happily boarded the airplane to go home to my beloved family.

As I entered the terminal in L.A., I saw my handsome Brad waiting for me. I ran to him and we hugged as if we'd been apart for years—a hug that rocketed to the tippy-top in the pantheon of Best Hugs of My Life. The entire two-hour drive home from L.A. to San Diego, we talked nonstop about my trip, though we had kept in constant contact throughout it. When I saw the girls at home, I dropped to my knees so I could hug them face-to-face, and they knocked me down, swarming me like excited puppies.

There's no place like home.

Chapter 46

In this new school year, there would be no nannies, no after-school programs, and no juggling schedules. Just Mommy.

Brad and I walked the girls to their first day of school. Second-grader Chloe was a ball of excited energy; fourth-grader Sophie was clinging to Brad's arm. Each, in her own way, was perfect. My girls had weathered the storm of the past year. This was a new beginning.

When I picked them up from school, they talked without taking a breath. They had so much to tell me! About their teachers! Their classmates! The books they were reading! At home, I made them a snack, since they were *starving*, and then it was time for homework. That evening, it was dinner as a family, a round of Crazy Eights, and then off to bed.

It was a simple life. A conventional life. A lovely life.

As the girls and I were walking to school the next morning, Chloe asked, "Mom, would you rather have a life that's short and fun or long and boring?"

Considering my recent head-to-head with the Grim Reaper, I was not eager to answer this question. And I wasn't all that excited to hear my seven-year-old pondering mortality, either.

"Long and fun," I evaded, wanting to change the subject.

Chloe bristled. "But you have to *choose*, Mommy." Her face was scrunched up and intense. She wasn't going to let me off the hook.

"Okay . . . short and fun," I relented. And it was the truth, if I had to pick.

Chloe smiled. That's what she had thought.

"Me too. Short and fun," she said. She didn't seem to understand the macabre nature of the conversation. To her, it was just a rhetorical exercise.

We shared a knowing smile.

And then Chloe and I both looked at Sophie. Sweet little Sophie. She looked sheepish.

Sophie shrugged her narrow shoulders, as if to say, *Okay, you got me.*

"Long and boring," she finally answered, with just a hint of apology in her voice.

But there was no need to be sorry. Sophie was perfectly Sophie.

Chapter 47

In November 2009—exactly one year since the start of chemo—I walked the red carpet at the Los Angeles Music Awards in Hollywood, amid flashbulbs and a flurry of questions from reporters. My album *Girl Like This* had been nominated for Country Album of the Year, and "Float Away" for Americana Single of the Year. It was mind-boggling.

I'd spent hours deciding what to wear—short dress, long dress, flowing or column? Sequins? Patterned? I finally settled on a floor-length, animal-print dress with an open back. I figured it was kind of rock-starry, but still classy. My hair was easy—I'd continued sporting a pixie length since treatment had ended. Just a little pomade, and I was good to go.

The Laura Roppé Band had been invited to perform "Float Away" during the show, and my entire band was buzzing. We were one of the last acts to perform, immediately following a Russian heavy-metal band, whose performance featured a clown makeup–clad lead singer, a children's choir, and a snow machine. (You know, I always find it most appealing to have my Russian-clown-metal music accompanied by children's voices and fake snow.)

Finally, as I stood at center stage, looking out at a room full of music-industry heavy hitters (whose ears were likely still ringing from the Russians before us), Jenny began playing the familiar opening chords of "Float Away" on her violin. I saw Brad's proud face in the audience, and my soul welled up, once again, with love for this man. Our lives had been turned upside down over the past year, and now it was time to savor our triumph.

And then, as I heard my voice rising up from my throat, wafting through the room, past the balcony seats and straight into the night sky, all the way up into the farthest reaches of heaven, where it shot like fireworks into a million little stars, all I could feel was peace: I was singing again, I was alive, and I had finally staked my claim on the life I'd always wanted to live. I could feel the audience's rapt attention. Perhaps they sensed they were witnessing a rebirth on that stage.

When they announced "Float Away" as the Americana Single of the Year, I wanted to collapse in a heap on the stage, as if I'd just reached the finish line of an arduous marathon. Luckily, Jennifer was standing there, too, as Instrumentalist of the Year, and she propped me up. We cried and laughed in each other's arms.

I was a jet-setter now, peeps!

I packed my bags for a week at the famed Rock 'n' Roll Fantasy Camp in Hollywood. I'd been invited by the camp's generous founder,

David Fishof, and sponsored by the angels at the breast cancer awareness organization Keep A Breast.

The gist of the camp was this: Musicians of any level came for a week. Campers were divided into bands of five or so people, led by a counselor—a musician with impressive credentials. Each "band" rehearsed daily for a big showcase to be held on the last day; meanwhile, big-name rock stars dropped in to wow everyone with their rock star–ness.

For a girl who loves music (and rock legends), it was heaven on Earth.

Upon my arrival, five other campers and I were assigned to a bighearted camp counselor known as Teddy Z, a keyboardist who'd toured with Guns N' Roses and Carole King, among others. Two of my new bandmates were successful entrepreneurs, two others had raided their savings to make their rock 'n' roll dreams a reality, and the fifth was an aw-shucks guy from Arkansas who'd won entry to the camp in a contest. And me? I was the wife-and-mother-of-two cancer survivor who was now a thirty-nine-year-old fledgling singer-songwriter. You know, the usual.

Not surprisingly, music made short shrift of our varied backgrounds, and almost instantly the members of my band became the best of friends.

On the first day of camp, I attended a songwriting class taught by Grammy-winning songwriter Mark Hudson, a larger-than-life personality who initially rose to fame in the '70s as part of the Hudson Brothers trio. In addition to having written some of the biggest radio hits, Hudson has produced records for big names like Aerosmith, Ringo

Starr, and Ozzy Osbourne. (And here's a fun fact for pop-culture junkies: Mark is also the uncle of the adorable actress Kate Hudson.)

As I settled into my chair at the workshop, spiral notebook in hand and ballpoint pen at the ready, I eagerly anticipated absorbing Mark's songwriting pearls of wisdom. Would it be "the top ten tricks to songwriting"? Or perhaps "how to write a hit song"? Either way, I was ready to take detailed notes.

But then Mark walked into the room, and I knew instantly this wasn't going to be your typical Learning Annex lecture. Maybe it was the fact that Mark was wearing a purple pimp suit. Or maybe it was his rainbow-streaked beard, which made him look as though he'd just taken first place in a rainbow pie–eating contest. Whatever it was, I knew this man was unlike anyone I'd ever met before. I was immediately transfixed.

"Hello," he said to his adoring audience of songwriting students. His eyes were fierce but warm.

"Hello," we answered back in unison.

"Hey, look, it's Guitar Zero," Mark proclaimed, motioning to one of the campers assigned to his fantasy band, a poor sap who'd apparently displayed less-than-stellar chops in their rehearsal earlier that day. "How're you doing?"

When the object of Mark's playful scorn bantered back that perhaps the real problem was Mark's leadership, not the camper's prowess as a guitar player, Mark laughed easily and heartily.

"Well, for some reason, they've asked me to speak to you all about songwriting," Mark began, turning his attention to the task at hand. "Ah, yes, one of my favorite topics."

I leaned forward in my seat, my eyes trained like lasers on his magnetic face. He seemed so comfortable in his own skin, so unapologetic.

"It's actually quite simple," he began. "The song has to tell *the truth*. Dig deep and find the truth." His voice rose with emotion. *"Always.* Or don't bother writing the song."

Someone in the audience asked a question then, but I didn't hear what the student said. The only person in the room, as far as I was concerned, was Mark Hudson. Everyone else had disappeared.

"Stand up and be yourself," Mark responded to the no-name pupil. "Be yourself, in your full glory, in your songwriting and in life. You can't write good songs if you aren't brave enough to be yourself."

I am certain I gasped. *You can't write good songs if you aren't brave enough to be yourself.* The words took my breath away.

Mark continued to tell some highly entertaining anecdotes about how he had written songs for Aerosmith, Celine Dion, Hanson, and others. And though I listened to every word, I could not move past his bone-crushing thesis: *You can't write good songs if you aren't brave enough to be yourself.*

After class, a crowd of fawning campers surrounded Mark, laughing, smiling, thanking him. They were jovial, backslapping. Merry.

I hung back, waiting for everyone else to leave the room. I was not merry. I couldn't breathe.

Finally Mark was alone and I approached, tears threatening to fill my eyes.

"Mark," I said. "Your words . . . " I could barely croak out the phrase. "Thank you" was all I managed. And then, dammit, tears began to distort my vision.

"You're welcome," he answered offhandedly, still glancing at the dissipating crowd. But then his eyes met mine and he saw the dark storm brewing beneath my contorted face. "Why are you so upset?" he asked, concerned.

"Oh, no, I'm not upset . . . I'm inspired. *I'm so inspired!*" And with that, those damned tears spilled out of my eyes and right down my cheeks. "I've never been so inspired in all my life!"

Mark looked relieved and touched. He smiled at me. He understood.

"Mark, would you mind listening to one of my songs?" I asked tentatively.

"I would *love* to," he answered, and his interest sounded genuine.

I was overjoyed. "Thank you so much, Mark," I said, fumbling in my purse for my CD. "Here you go. Thank you! Track three: 'Float Away'!"

That night, I tossed and turned, imagining *the* Mark Hudson actually listening to a song of *mine*. I just couldn't get over the idea of him listening to *my voice!* What if he liked it? But what if didn't? What if he hated it? What if he told me I shouldn't quit my day job?

The next morning, after waiting for yet another doting crowd to clear out from around Mark, I approached him at the bagels-and-cream-cheese table.

"Good morning," I said, trying not to seem like a pest, trying to seem like I was only vaguely interested in whether he'd listened to the song.

"Ah, yes, good morning," he answered, as he poured himself a cup of coffee. "I slept with you last night, you know," he said. And then, to my expectant face, he explained, "I fell asleep listening to your album, on my third time through."

I clapped my hands together involuntarily in the universal sign of "oh, goodie!" He had listened to my *entire album?* And *more than once?!*

"I couldn't stop listening," he continued. "*Your voice!* I could feel you in each song."

I had goose bumps! The great Mark Hudson had *felt* me in each song!

"But, Laura, you need to keep going," he encouraged, looking at me with those piercing eyes and grabbing my full attention. "You're on the right path. You, my dear, are a songwriter. But you were holding back in these songs, both as a songwriter and as a vocalist. You're just trying too damned hard to be perfect and pretty, honey. There's so much more to you than that. I *know* there's more inside of you! Now go find it. Go deeper. Be willing to fail. Don't get bogged down in trying to do it *right*. Songwriting isn't about being *right;* it's about being *real.*"

I was blown away. He had hit the nail on the head. I nodded my assent, at a loss for words.

"Be willing to fail," he said, his tone gentle, "and I promise you will soar to great heights."

Mark was right. I had been holding back, afraid to fail. In my songs. And in life. The songs on my album—all written when I cared what others thought of me, before I'd fully committed to following my heart, back when I'd been afraid that people might call me a "dreamer," before I'd been ravaged by cancer and forced to own the deepest truths about myself—were not as vulnerable, as real, as the songs I'd been writing since my treatments. Mark Hudson was right: It was time to let go and expose myself in all my flawed glory—both in life and in my songs.

I felt that familiar electric current coursing through my body: *I have to record a second album.*

The next day at camp, famed Kiss guitarist Ace Frehley talked to us about some of his musical adventures. After his group question-and-answer session, I managed to chat briefly with him one-on-one.

"You can have a big house with maids and a garage full of cars," he told me in his tough-guy voice, straight out of *Goodfellas,* "but you gotta be inspired every day, or it's all nothin'."

I nodded. I hadn't expected Ace Frehley to be so deep.

The next day, Meat Loaf walked into our rehearsal room in the middle of a song. When we had finished, he beelined over to me.

"You need to *own* it," he counseled me urgently. His eyes were aflame. "*This is your stage.* Don't hold back! You're holding back!" He raised his arms in a dramatic flourish to emphasize his point.

"Thank you . . . Meat Loaf." *Mr. Meat Loaf? Mr. Loaf?* "I'm . . . yes . . . Thank you. Will do."

It was surreal. I was getting performance advice from Meat Loaf! The original bat out of hell! And he was beating the same drum I'd been hearing all week: I was holding back.

Okay, okay, Universe! I hear you loud and clear!

It was time to let go, to expose myself, to take a flying-squirrel leap with all my heart. It was time to go bare-assed in the display window at Macy's.

The next day, the camp welcomed Jon Anderson, the wildly talented front man and songwriter for Yes. You know, "Owner of a Lonely Heart"? (And now you have that song stuck in your head, don't you?)

Before Mr. Anderson's arrival, we campers were warned not to get too touchy-feely with this particular rock star. Admire him without touching, we were told—hugging, hand shaking, and groping were no-no's. Apparently, Mr. Anderson had recently been felled by a nasty flu, and, understandably, he'd grown leery of being pawed by his germy, though adoring, public. Adoration: good. Germs: bad.

And then, only a few minutes after the enunciation of Mr. Anderson's "no-germ policy," there he was: blond hair, boyish face, unassuming and gentle demeanor. He reacted to our boisterous applause with a crooked smile and a wave, and we all settled into our chairs in anticipation of a camp-wide question-and-answer session.

Much to the thrill of the audience, Mr. Anderson picked up an acoustic guitar and performed an angelic, simple version of "Starship Trooper," for which everyone gave him a standing ovation. His iconic voice was pure and without pretense.

The hair on my arms stood on end as I listened. *This is exactly what Mark Hudson was talking about,* I said to myself as I applauded enthusiastically. *I understand.*

"Thank you so much," Mr. Anderson said humbly. "Thank you."

And with that, the question-and-answer session disassembled and we campers separated back into our individual bands for further rehearsals.

Just as I was singing my heart out in my band's rehearsal room,

Mr. Anderson entered the room. After watching for a moment, on a whim, he walked over to a spare microphone and began singing backup to my lead vocals.

Jon Anderson is my backup singer!

My singing quickly devolved into a sort of singsong laughter—the sound that comes out of someone experiencing unadulterated glee.

At the end of our spontaneous joint performance, Mr. Anderson approached me, smiling. "I like your voice," he said, and I blushed.

Don't touch him, I reminded myself. *Germs: bad.*

"Thank you," I responded to his kindness, taking a careful step back. "I'm actually a fledgling songwriter," I told him. "Could you please share any songwriting advice?" I looked at him hopefully, careful to keep my germs at a distance.

Jon Anderson assessed me, a relaxed, earnest smile on his lips, and then took a bold step toward me, right into my personal space (and into the zone of optimum airborne-illness transmission). And then, much to my shock, he grasped my shoulders and gazed straight into my face. "I see you," he said. "You are beautiful. Just let the songs come through you. Don't stop to think; just let them come through you. Just let the world see exactly what I see right now."

Our eyes were locked for a moment, his hands pressed firmly against my shoulders. Words wouldn't form, so I collapsed into him and hugged him, a surge of emotion overcoming me.

He hugged me right back, tenderly, sweetly.

When we pulled apart, he nodded his head and whispered, "Namaste." And then he waved to everyone and left the room.

It took me over an hour to fully regain my composure.

On the last day of Rock 'n' Roll Fantasy Camp, campers and counselors alike trekked over to the Whisky a Go Go, where each band would perform a camp-closing set of songs. Déjà vu flooded me as I walked through the door of the Whisky and onto the floor adjacent to the stage: It had been twenty years since I had stood in exactly the same spot with Amy Bo Bamy and Marco, clutching my sides with laughter at the sight of Val Kilmer's pirouetting dance double. Twenty years! Where had the time gone?

"Laura, we're up," my bandmate called to me, and I was startled back to the present. It was time for us to make rock history, baby!

I followed my bandmates up one flight of stairs to the balcony, across the dilapidated upstairs viewing area, and then down another flight of back steps leading to stage access. After exchanging high fives and "break a leg"s with my band, I stepped out onto the Whisky stage and right down to front and center, to the precise square inch of real estate that had been calling my name for twenty years.

This was the *exact spot* where the iconic Jim Morrison had performed "The End" forty years before, and where Val Kilmer had *simulated* the iconic Jim Morrison performing "The End" twenty years before, right in front of my nineteen-year-old, starstruck eyes. This was the very coordinate on Planet Earth I had lusted to occupy as I'd watched Val Kilmer writhing around in his black leather pants—back when I'd been certain that my jaw-dropping performance as Girl One would rocket me to superstardom.

And now here I was, not quite the superstar I had once envisioned, but a thirty-nine-year-old woman, wife, and mother of two—a survivor who'd been to the hinterlands of hell and back.

And I was standing on the Whisky stage, at long last, ready to claim my long-awaited moment in the spotlight.

And what song was I slated to perform that night at the Whisky? None other than the Doors' classic "Love Me Two Times"! On top of that, in one of those instances that beg the question whether "coincidences" exist, the mystery rock star joining my band on guitar that night, arranged by the camp, was none other than Robby Krieger himself, the real-life legendary guitarist for the Doors.

I had fallen into a wormhole.

I looked over at Robby's mellow face and nodded my head—*let's do it*—and he started playing the familiar guitar introduction to "Love Me Two Times." My heart was thumping in my ears and my head was spinning. And, yes, of course, my hands were shaking, too.

I'm pretty sure I flubbed the lyrics to the song (which takes a written book of instructions to do, simple and iconic as it is), though it's all a blur now, and I'd be surprised if I was on pitch more than half the song. But, of course, I was enthralled during every second of the performance. It was truly a rock 'n' roll fantasy.

As I climbed up the steps leading off the stage and onto the balcony, Mark Hudson was waiting for me at the top.

"You did good, kid," he said. And then he shot me a beautiful, wide smile, framed perfectly by his rainbow-colored beard.

Walking through my front door after arriving home from Rock 'n' Roll Fantasy Camp, I instantly began yammering breathlessly to Brad about every detail of my week. Mark Hudson!

Meat Loaf! Ace Frehley! Jon Anderson! I thanked him for holding down the fort yet again, and for allowing me to gallivant through yet another exciting adventure. And then, finally, after I'd exhausted every last anecdote about my week in la-la land, I dropped the bomb: "Babe, I've decided I absolutely *must* record another album." I paused for effect. *"Right now."*

I waited for Brad to resist. To roll his eyes and wonder aloud why I had to go so . . . *big* with all of this. But he didn't. In fact, he didn't seem surprised at all. "Of course you do, honey," he responded. "Lucy's gotta get into the Copacabana."

I kissed Brad, laughing, and rushed to make a phone call to the person who had opened the front door of my tornado-ravaged, black-and-white house, the person who had allowed me to see how colorful life could be if only I would reveal, and embrace, my true heart.

Matthew sounded happy to hear from me, as usual.

"Hey, Cuz," he greeted me in his familiar, laid-back voice. "How's it going?"

"Hey, Cuz," I answered back, smiling into the phone. "I've decided to make my second album."

"Naturally."

"Will you produce it for me?" I knew it was a lot to ask, given his busy touring schedule.

"Cuz, I thought you'd never ask."

Chapter 48

When I was lying in bed—bald, skinny, and gray, not sure if I was still alive or if my ship had already sailed—I heard a soft voice whispering in my ear. *You'll thank me one day,* it said.

In my vulnerable and weakened state, I was not surprised to hear the voice, actually, but I *was* surprised by the content of the message. How could I ever be thankful for this nightmare? *Cancer is a bastard. May it never come back into my life, and may it never be visited on another human being.*

And yet here I am, two years past my initial diagnosis, and there is no doubt that cancer has been the catalyst for untold blessings in my life. And for those blessings, I do indeed say thank you.

For one thing, were it not for cancer, I never would have known that my face shape is so well suited to short hair. *Thank you, cancer!*

But, of course, there's more to be thankful for than a flattering new hairstyle. Much more.

I now have the inside scoop about a card game being played every single day right under our noses: Every day, God fans out a deck of cards, facedown, and instructs: *Pick a card, any card.* Until I picked the "cancer card" that fateful day, my card had always read PICK ANOTHER CARD. And I had just taken that for granted. When I eventually pulled the card with CANCER stamped across it, I cursed my bad luck. I felt singled out. *This must be a mistake!* But then, slowly, with time and lots of support, I accepted my card. And, with no other option, I played the card I had been dealt to the best of my ability.

Now, I know I must go "all in" with my chips, every single day. I can't control anything else, perhaps, but I can choose to be happy right now. And if I make that choice, then that's everything. Because only *right now* actually exists, anyway. I'm just grateful for every day I get to pick a card.

Thank you, cancer.

I was stripped bare by cancer, and I'm not talking about losing my hair or my hips (which have both come back, by the way). Losing my physical self somehow jump-started the process of losing extra figurative baggage, too. As I battled for my very life, it took too much energy to nurture any pretenses, and the layers started peeling off, one by one, until I was exposed and raw. Off went my vanity. Goodbye, ego. Adios, people-pleasing. Sayonara, complacency. Arrivederci, pride. And then, at the bitter end, my self-confidence and self-reliance left me, too. I was completely humbled and in need.

When my treatments were over and some color had come back into my cheeks, I turned my attention to all those layers crumpled in a heap on the floor. And I realized, *Hey, I can cherry-pick which ones to put back on.* First things first: I quickly picked up and reattached my newly refurbished self-confidence and self-reliance. *Whew!* And then I examined everything else in the pile. *Hmm.* There was nothing else worth reattaching, so I left everything else on the floor.

In all that new space, my true self expanded, flooding into nooks and crannies my cast-offs had previously occupied. I was a helium balloon, filled to the brim with who I really am. Life became . . . simpler.

I do not pretend to have spiritual or medical answers for anyone else, but I believe that the mind, body, and spirit are all connected. For many years, I thought I could wear a colorful scarf around my neck, despite the fact that scarves are not me at all, and play a character in a movie constructed inside my head, without consequences for my soul. I thought I could do all the "right things," the things a good person is "supposed to do"—unrelated to my deepest hopes and desires and talents—and nonetheless feel sufficiently fulfilled in life by external kudos and approval. I thought I could live with extreme stress at my job for the majority of my waking hours, forcing myself to be a pit bull when I wasn't one—and yet not have that stress affect my mind, body, or spirit. I thought I could *compartmentalize.*

Well, we all know how that worked out for me. By day I felt physically ill, like I had a "terminal illness"; and by night I dodged oncoming locomotives. And yet I never changed course—until the day I was diagnosed with cancer. Really, I would have saved myself a lot of aggravation if I'd just listened to (and followed) my inner voice before it began shrieking hysterically into my ear. Within *minutes* of learning I'd been diagnosed with cancer, I was defiantly declaring the end of my legal career. Why the hell did I think I needed the golden ticket of a potentially terminal illness to begin living my life in earnest?

Before cancer, I had started down the path of self-emancipation, of course. I had already recorded my album and was happily skipping down the musical road. But I was doing so with caution. "I'm a lawyer who sings," I told people at cocktail parties, enjoying the novelty but not wanting to be pegged as a full-blown "dreamer." Were it not for cancer (or perhaps some other life-changing event that might have come along), it is highly unlikely, in my view, that I would have taken a belly-flopping leap of faith—a leap with all my heart—to pursue my dreams. I probably would have stayed grounded in my head, at least in part, never willing to admit to the world at large, "Yes, my head is in the clouds. I follow my heart. Oh, and by the way, I'm a people person, too."

As it turns out, when I have faith in myself, when I listen carefully to the voice inside me, I am my own best woobie.

It has been quite some time since I dreamed my bare ass was the main attraction at Macy's or that a train was barreling through my bedroom. Have I finally conquered my lifelong anxieties? I'm getting there—though, in the interest of full disclosure, Brad says I still occasionally demand in my sleep, "Who the hell are you?" Apparently, I'm still working on it. But I am grateful for my progress.

Thank you, cancer.

And here's something else I am sure about, now more than ever, thanks to cancer: Nothing is insurmountable. One day, we will all die. (I'm sorry if I just spoiled the ending for you.) Dying is the worst that can happen, right? That being the case, there can be no permanent downside to striving to optimize one's self, to at least trying to live one's dreams. I now understand: There is no permanent downside to being the real me, to opening my heart and exposing myself to pain. Because pain is not permanent. But regret is. And, of course, the upside to trying all of these things is limitless.

When I was at UCLA, I took an ancient-Greek philosophy class that has stayed with me all these years; in particular, I've never forgotten Plato's "Allegory of the Cave." Forgive me if I butcher this, but this is how I remember it from twenty years ago: There is a group of men living in a cave, all shackled together in a row. They were born there, and they've never left. Year after year, the shackled men sit, bound together, staring at the wall of the cave. Just behind them, where they cannot see, there is a bonfire that throws shadows onto the wall in front of the men. The bound men are entranced by the flickering shadows on the wall.

One day, a man at the end of the row breaks free of his chains. Once freed, he turns around and sees the bonfire and realizes the source of the shadows he's watched his whole life. He tries to convince the others of what he sees, but they do not believe him.

"Let's leave this place! Let's see what else is out there!" the freed man exclaims.

"There is nothing more than this," the others say.

But the freed man will not be deterred. He makes his way to the mouth of the cave and steps outside for the first time. He is overcome by a blinding light—the glorious sun! At first his eyes are pained by the brightness of the light and by the vibrant colors he has never witnessed before. But soon he is able to adjust to his new surroundings. And, he realizes, they're beautiful. He exults. He races back to share his discovery with the shackled men.

"You must come! There is much more than this outside the cave!"

But the shackled men, who have never left the cave, cannot conceive of a world outside it. They have no way to fathom the sun. They are content to watch the shadows flickering on the cave wall. It's all they know.

I apologize to you if you are a certified Greek philosopher. But this rendition, whether accurate or not, is what has stayed with me all these years. The moment I read this allegory at age nineteen, I knew I didn't want to be one of the shackled men in the dim cave, watching shadows flicker on a wall. I wanted to venture outside into the bright sunlight, even if it meant initially searing my eyes. And yet, despite this innate yearning inside me, there were times in my life when I settled for dim light and flickering shadows, out of fear or complacency. *It's comfortable here,* I told myself. *This is just fine.*

Now, though, I know I must never stop searching for the bright light outside the cave. I must strive to learn and explore, and to stretch myself in ways I have not thought possible. And I must do so in ways that are true to me. Rather than being maniacally driven to *accomplish*, I must take greater care in choosing *what* to accomplish.

As with the freed man in Plato's cave, my shackles have clanked to the ground, and I have turned around to behold the flickering bonfire behind me. And do you know what I have seen in the illusory flames? My need for others' approval. My lifelong willingness to let others define me. My pursuit of "success" without regard to personal cost. My overblown sense of my own importance. Shadows of reality.

And when I ventured outside the cave, do you know what I witnessed there? Love. Powerful, healing, nothing-else-matters, lift-me-up, wipe-my-tears-away love. Higher love from God (or the universe or the collective conscience) that has the power to uplift and heal! Love from strangers, my new brothers and sisters! Love from family, my dearest ones, the keepers of my heart, whom I will never take for granted again! Love for myself—my flawed, big-dreaming, optimistic, spaztastic, late-blooming, adventure-loving, bighearted self! Love is the light I saw when I ventured outside the cave. There was nothing else out there. Or if there was, I didn't see it.

One of the first things people want to know when they talk to me now is, "Did chemo work?" I know everyone wants to hear me say, "Abso-fricking-lutely!" I hate to disappoint people, I really do, but the honest answer is, "Who the hell knows?" The surgeon took out the initial tumor and lymph nodes, and I choose to believe that no cancer cells remained after that. Of course, if my optimism is wrong and bastard cancer cells did remain after surgery, then I am certain chemo blasted every single rogue cell to kingdom come—and then poisoned, nuked, stabbed, shot, karate-chopped, and electrocuted them, just for good measure.

I will officially be in remission in three more years, when I hit my five-year mark without a problem. Until then, how do I know if it "worked" or not? I just have to wait and see. But I refuse to spend the next three years waiting to cross some imaginary finish line. I'm just going to live my life to its fullest in the here and now.

Remember when Dorothy, trapped in the Wicked Witch's tower, watched in terror as the grains of sand fell unabated into the bottom half of the hourglass? Even as a child, I couldn't help but wonder why Dorothy just sat there, staring at the hourglass. Why didn't she check to see if the tower door was, by some lucky chance, unlocked? Or maybe look for a secret passageway? She could have used her time so much more wisely!

If you knew the Wicked Witch had turned over an hourglass to mark the end of your life, would you sit in the tower, fretting and staring at the grains of falling sand? Or, with whatever time was left, would you beat down that damned tower door, bitch-slap a flying monkey or two, and move on down the road? Speaking for myself, I'm gonna bitch-slap the monkeys and boogie on down the Yellow Brick Road.

Epilogue

After my return from Rock 'n' Roll Fantasy
Camp at the end of 2009, Matthew and I immediately began recording my second album throughout 2010. Each time he came home for a
few weeks from a leg of his world tour, we disappeared into the studio
together for days at a time.

Oftentimes, our sides hurt from laughing so hard; occasionally,
perhaps inspired by our mutual brilliance at capturing a perfect drum
solo or slide-guitar lick, we danced around the studio together like
Kevin Bacon and Chris Penn in *Footloose*. Many times, despite our
best intentions, recording never happened on a particular day, and
instead we spent our time together sitting in the studio, talking, hugging, and crying away the hours. But mostly we just enjoyed the thrill
of creating music together, the joy of sharing our common passion.

At the end of that year, despite Matt's crazy touring schedule and
my own frantic schedule as a wife and mother of two busy girls (sports

for Sophie and musical theater for Chloe), Matthew and I managed to bring my songs to life. And oh, the joy! They turned out exactly as I'd envisioned.

It was a magical year. It was the year I found, and revealed, my true voice.

Not surprisingly, then, it was also the year I wrote this book.

Whenever Matt went off on another leg of his tour, temporarily halting progress on the album and leaving me pent up with unfulfilled artistic energy, I quenched my creative thirst by arranging words on my computer screen for hours at a time. Every night after I put the girls to sleep, and after Brad's rhythmic breathing next to me confirmed he'd drifted off into dreamland, I crept to my computer and wrote, and wrote, and wrote, usually until the wee hours of the morning.

And whenever Matt came home, I swapped my nighttime writing sessions for recording sessions with him.

Thus, throughout that year, the two projects—the book and the album—became indistinguishable to me, two means of telling the same story simultaneously.

When I released my second album in early 2011, which I christened *I'm Still Here* (complete with a back-cover photograph of my badass tattoo), I held my breath, eager to find out if the world would hear the new clarity in my voice. And if people did hear it, would they like it?

I got my answer soon enough: A respected music blog called my album "a brilliant and emotionally naked artistic turn" and applauded its "startling emotional honesty."

And then *Billboard* magazine, a truly iconic music publication, ranked me number three on its list of the top fifty emerging artists in the world. Not too shabby for a forty-year-old (former) lawyer, wife, and mother of two! And it got even better: For twenty weeks following my initial entry onto the Billboard chart, I remained there, bouncing around, week after glorious week.

"I feel like a proud father," Mark Hudson said when he called to congratulate me on my album, which I'd sent to him with an effusive thank-you note. "You did it, Laura! *You did it.* It's a masterpiece."

But before I could get too full of myself, he added, "Now, Laura, it's time to go even further. I know you've got even more inside you!"

And, of course, he was right.

Acknowledgments

This book's existence has depended on the support and generosity of some very special people. At the top of the list is Brad, my woobie and my rock. Let's face it: Your memorable zingers throughout the years have supplied half the content of this book. And my lovely little girls deserve so much credit, too. Sophie, in particular: You peeked over my shoulder the entire time I wrote this book (except when I told you to go away because I was writing something intended for "mature audiences"), and your exclamations of "Mommy, you are such a good writer!" and "Mommy, you are so funny!" kept me going and believing in myself. Even when you were ten years old, I trusted your judgment that much, honey. Chloe, my little stick of dynamite: Keep dreaming, keep singing, keep writing, keep strutting your stuff, little mama. Thank you so much for your great idea that led me directly to the title of this book!

Jane Barker, My Dearest Jane, my chemo buddy and soul sister, thank you for holding my hand from across the pond. Allyson

Aabram, you read and reread every draft of this book and pushed me to reveal more and more. Thank you. Dad, you can see what I see, even when it's crazy! I love you, Pops. Jill Marr, thank you for believing in me and changing my life. Sharon, words on a page aren't enough. You know what you mean to me. Mom, thank you for calling me Lamby when I was little. Matthew, you showed me who I could be. Lorlou, you inspired me to be a writer. Thanks and acknowledgment to my entire family for their boundless love and support.

Thank you to the wonderful folks at Seal Press, especially my editor, the generous and spirited Brooke Warner. Special acknowledgment and heartfelt thanks to Andrew Hampshire, Paula Dozzi, Lesley Ballard, Cristina Almeida, my CBL brothers, JR Reed, Jack Black, Mark Hudson, Triple Negative Breast Cancer Foundation, Jennifer Griffin, Amanda Nixon, Kimmy McAtee, Keep A Breast, David Fishof, Beverly Trainer, Caroline and Emil Wohl, Tommy Sablan and the Jeff & Jer team, Wildy Haskell, the folks at Right Recordings, Jennifer Argenti, Leslie Tall Manning, Martha Lawrence, Lisa Pulitzer, Joni Rodgers, the Bogans, the Zamoyskis, Tiffanie Kasner, Heather Dugdale, and, of course, The Bunco Girls. And to those of you mentioned throughout this book: I'm a better person for having known you (or, in some instances, having dreamed of knowing you).

About the Author

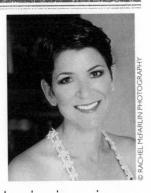

Laura Roppé is an award-winning singer-songwriter, cancer survivor, speaker, and former attorney from San Diego, California. She obtained a BA in theater arts from UCLA (summa cum laude) but then pursued the "family business" by attending law school at the University of San Diego, where she graduated number two in her class, and went on to practice employment/business litigation for over a decade.

In 2008, the year of her diagnosis with triple negative breast cancer at age thirty-seven, Laura ditched her legal career to follow her musical dreams in earnest, winning Americana Single of the Year at the 2009 Los Angeles Music Awards. Upon the release of Laura's second album, *I'm Still Here,* which she wrote during chemo treatments, *Billboard* magazine ranked her number three on its chart of the top fifty emerging artists in the world. Laura spends her time with her husband, two daughters, and dog, Buster; writes and sings; plays bunco on the second Tuesday of every month with her girlfriends; and, last but not least, devises various schemes to get herself into the Copacabana. For more information, go to www.lauraroppe.com.

Selected Titles from Seal Press

For more than thirty years, Seal Press has published groundbreaking books. By women. For women.

Marrying George Clooney: Confessions from a Midlife Crisis, by Amy Ferris. $16.95, 978-1-58005-297-9. In this candid look at menopause, Amy Ferris chronicles every one of her funny, sad, hysterical, down and dirty, and raw to the bones insomnia-fueled stories.

Another Morning: Voices of Truth and Hope From Mothers With Cancer, by Linda Blachman. $15.95, 978-1-58005-178-1. A collection of powerful, inspirational, and deeply moving personal stories of ordinary women responding to every mother's nightmare: a cancer diagnosis while raising children.

Lessons from the Monk I Married, by Katherine Jenkins. $15.00, 978-1-58005-368-6. Katherine Jenkins offers up ten powerful lessons about life, love, and spirituality that she has gathered during her marriage to former Buddhist monk Seong Yoon Lee.

Something Spectacular: The True Story of One Rockette's Battle with Bulimia, by Greta Gleissner. $17.00, 978-1-58005-415-7. A piercing, powerful account of one woman's struggle with bulimia, self-image, and sexuality, set against the backdrop of professional dancing.

A Thousand Sisters: My Journey into the Worst Place on Earth to Be a Woman, by Lisa Shannon, foreword by Zainab Salbi. $16.95, 978-1-58005-359-4. Through her inspiring story of turning what started as a solo 30-mile run to raise money for Congolese women into a national organization, Run for Congo Women, Lisa Shannon sounds a deeply moving call to action for each person to find in them the thing that brings meaning to a wounded world.

Follow My Lead: What Training My Dogs Taught Me about Life, Love, and Happiness, by Carol Quinn. $17.00, 978-1-58005-370-9. Unhappy with her failing love affair, her stagnant career, and even herself, Carol Quinn enrolls her two Rhodesian ridgebacks into dog agility training—and becomes the "alpha dog" of her own life in the process.

Find Seal Press Online

www.SealPress.com
www.Facebook.com/SealPress
Twitter: @SealPress